WHY ME?

The *unfair* reason you get cavities and what to do about it.

1st Edition

DR. V. KIM KUTSCH,

ISBN: 978-0-000000-0

Printed by Select Impressions in the United States of America.

Cover design by Alana Rodrigues
Book design by www.PAZ.Design

First printing edition, 2020

Soapbox Publishing
11959 Sunrise Plateau Dr.
Anacortes WA, 98221

www.carifree.com

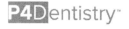

This book is dedicated to Bob Bowers,

who still inspires us to do what we think is best

each and every day.

Contents

FOREWORD

Why Me? is a much needed book intended for dental patients who want to know why they get cavities and how to cure themselves of this disease so they never again suffer from cavities. Cleverly written with useful tools, this book will leave you asking: "Why not me? Because I now have the tools to be cavity-free forever." Although this book is intended for patients, not all healthcare providers understand the material presented in this book and I recommend it be read by all professionals treating this disease. It should be utilized with every patient as an integral part of every dental office. It sends the clear message that improving oral health will improve overall health. In fact, it may even save your life! This book will empower patients to take control of their fate and search out a dental provider that will use these science-based methods. It will help force change to a system that will make them healthier. Ask "Why not?"

Douglas A. Young, DDS, EdD, MBA, MS

This is a very unique book that balances the science of why you get cavities with informative and simplified content that is clear and easy to understand. In order to accomplish this, Dr. Kim Kutsch has orchestrated a series of patient scenarios that allows us to move from passive observer to active investigator, making the reader more engaged and capable of determining why they may have cavities. You will realize that the overly simplistic explanation of "brushing after meals and stop eating sweets" is not enough to help those that are susceptible to this disease. Therefore, this book will, for the first time, allow the reader to determine their own multi-factorial reasons for their cavities and become able to understand how to prevent them from ever occurring in the future. Anyone that has ever had a cavity should read this book.

John C. Kois, DMD, MSD

INTRODUCTION

Why Read This Book?

We all grew up learning some basics about cavities: if you brush and floss as your dentist says, you should be cavity-free. Well, as you know, it isn't that easy. I am sure you or someone you know has followed your dentist's advice to the T yet still has a mouth full of fillings.

I have been working with people just like you for more than forty years. They brush and floss and still spend thousands of dollars and countless hours in the dental office. I am an expert in cariology (the study of dental caries or cavities) and have spent my career teaching dentists across the globe what I've learned. After all my years working with patients and studying dental cavities, I am shocked by the myths still circulating—and the misinformation about how to heal or reverse decay. I am also stunned by how much we learn each year about how our teeth are directly connected to the functions of the rest of our bodies. My goal with this book is to reshape how the public views cavities, to bust some of the old myths, and to give everyone some solid steps to take to prevent and limit the future risk for decay. In all honesty, I want this resource to be the beginning of the conversation. The real goal is not to determine how many cavities you have but to stop and ask why you have cavities in the first place. If we can figure that out, we have a chance for you to become healthy. As a grandfather, I want my grandkids to be part of a cavity-free generation, and that can start with us.

How to Use This Book

Dentists (me included) have struggled to figure out the best way to talk to patients about cavities. It is easy to overcomplicate the information, as the disease process is quite complex. When we do this, we tend to lose our patients' interest. You are busy people, and reading the latest study published in the *Journal of the American Dental Association* probably isn't high on your priority list. Most dentists have fallen into the trap of oversimplifying the information to keep the conversation quick and to the point—unfortunately, when doctors do this, patients don't fully understand their disease. I hope this book strikes a good balance between the academic and the everyday, between simple and educational. I have written the book in a way that values your time and your intelligence. It is intended to be a quick reference and a smart and useful resource. Each chapter begins with a real-life patient story you may be able to relate to, followed by an overview of the content, so you can easily skim the page to see what might best apply to you. My hope is you find everything helpful in some way, and that you also gather the information in an order that best applies to your situation, to be able to answer the question, why me?

Dental caries, the disease that causes cavities, is the number one disease of humankind. This is true for every country and every demographic in each country. It's a complex disease to diagnose and treat, and it can be frustrating for dental professionals and patients alike. It's pretty straightforward to repair a cavity with a filling or a crown, but getting to the root cause of the cavity is more challenging—so much so, that the decay rate continues to grow, and the oral health burden from cavities has remained unchanged. If it was as simple as a roll of floss and some fluoride, there would be no need for this book. But it's more complicated than that. My goal here is to break this disease down to its basics and simplify it so you can determine what's causing your cavities, fix the problem, and stop getting cavities.

Throughout each chapter I highlight sections using these symbols:

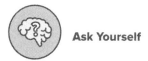

Ask Yourself

Cavities, you will learn, are in large part regulated by your behavior. Throughout the book, there will be times when you can ask yourself if certain things apply to your life. If so, there will be specific recommendations and information for you.

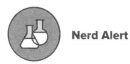

Nerd Alert

As I mentioned, I am an expert in cariology, which means I read all the scientific studies and rub elbows with many of the researchers in the field. If there is a scientific term or resource I use to explain a point, I will warn you before doing so.

Take Action

The point of this book is to help all of us change our understanding and our behavior. However, when learning something new, it can be hard to know exactly what to do and when to do it. I will provide action steps throughout the book that have worked well for my patients over the years.

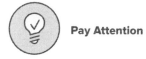

Pay Attention

I know your time is limited. If you are able to skim the information in this book, look for the light bulbs. I will provide quick tips; if nothing else, these will help you understand cavities a bit better and help you move toward better health.

Now that we have the symbols covered and you know a little bit about me, let's dig into the good stuff!

A Different Way to Think about Your Oral Health

Really taking control of your oral health requires more than just a better understanding of how caries disease works. It involves rethinking how you interact with your health and your health-care team. Just like drilling out a cavity and filling it with replacement material does not solve caries disease, visiting the dentist once you have symptoms that worry you about the condition of your teeth is no way keep your mouth healthy. It's a reactive way to handle your health instead of a proactive way to approach your health.

Caries Risk Assessment is a proactive tool to help manage your oral health. If you are committed to working with your dental care team to manage your risk and seek a cavity-free future, you will need to be part of a team that takes a different approach to managing your health. There is an established model called P4 Medicine that, when applied to dentistry, helps build a team approach to proactively keep you healthy.

The Four P's of taking care of your health in this new way include:

1. Predictive
2. Preventive
3. Personalized
4. Participatory

Let's take a look at each one in a little more detail so we can understand how this works.

Predictive

The predictive part stresses knowing illness early, well before serious symptoms have the chance to develop. It may mean screening for genetic risk factors. It may mean learning what the earliest possible symptoms look like before any symptoms or problems develop, which lets everyone on the medical team prepare for a possible problem before it even starts. Predictive medicine stresses preparing for a problem before there is a problem. It also uses knowledge about your current health to predict your likely future health.

Preventive

Preventive goes hand in hand with predictive. The only thing better for your health than being able to predict how likely you are to have a problem is having the tools to prevent the potential problem from becoming an actual problem. Even if it is not possible to stop a problem from starting, the preventive part of P4 Dentistry™ model lets you and your health-care team recognize early signs of illnesses so you can prevent serious illnesses or health issues. After all, the goal of prevention is to help you enjoy a healthy future, rather than a life of managed chronic illness.

Personalized

What's better than a custom-made dress shirt, perfectly tailored to your specific measurements? The answer is a custom-made health management plan that allows you to have the very best care and live your life in the very best daily health possible. The P4 health-care model focuses on wellness and on using personalized treatments and planning for each individual, and dental care is no different in this model from other medical care. You can focus on staying well instead of trying to get better from conditions or illnesses that could have been prevented. You are a unique individual, and a one-size-fits-all approach to health-care does not fit anybody well.

Participatory

P4 Dentistry™ model gives you power to help direct your health care. The participatory part lets you make better health-care decisions for yourself by keeping you informed about your conditions, your risks, and your options to control any possible conditions. You are fully part of the health-care team, participating in decisions about how to handle your health. Of course you are obligated to learn about your health. Doing so means you can make educated decisions about it, enabling the P4 model to work for you. Reading books like this one can be a great help as you seek to become a well-informed part of your own medical team.

How does the P4 Dentistry™ model relate to your goal of living cavity-free?

As we look at caries disease in this book, we will be looking at the big picture. We will look at the potential causes, the early, subtle signs that the disease process has begun, and the factors, both genetic and behavioral, that influence how likely you are to develop caries disease. These predictive factors help you identify which preventive steps are most likely to help you control the caries process. I want you to have confidence to work with your dental health team to create a personalized plan for your daily oral care and participate in your treatment strategy so you can get the most for your personal health and well-being.

As we look at specific risk factors and treatments throughout this book, we'll take this opportunity to point out how the P4 Dentistry model fits into a caries treatment plan and how to be a better-informed patient, active in your own medical care.

PART ONE:

The Science of Cavities

Chapter 1

Why Me?
Treating Cavities like
a Game of Whack-a-Mole

Have I had a cavity in the last year?

Do I brush and floss like a pro but still get cavities?

Am I frustrated with how many cavities I or someone in my family is getting?

Ask Yourself *If you answered YES to any of the above questions, this chapter is especially for you!*

IN THIS CHAPTER:

■ Cavities are caused by a disease, known as dental caries, which is an imbalance of your biofilm (sticky layer of bacteria and microbes on your teeth).

■ Five things can contribute to your risk of this dysfunction:
1. Lack of saliva
2. Diet
3. Bacteria (biofilm microbes)
4. Genetics
5. pH

■ The imbalance cannot be cured by filling the cavity.

■ This is about much more than your teeth.

Cavities Are a Sign of Something Bigger

I'll never forget Helen. She had been a patient of mine for many years. Early in our relationship I restored all of her old and broken fillings with expensive crowns and gold inlays. When we were finished, she had strong, beautiful, healthy teeth. For the next fifteen years or so, she didn't have a single cavity. She and her husband were dairy farmers and lived a healthy lifestyle. Then one year she missed her annual checkup. I should add that we live in the Willamette Valley of Oregon, famous for its Pinot Noir wines now, but it has always been the grass seed capital of the world. I proudly grew up on a grass seed farm myself. The valley is covered in acres of beautiful green grass fields. It's truly a magical place. The only downside is that when the grasses pollinate in the spring, the pollen count makes life diffi-cult for people with allergies. Some people, like Helen, develop those allergies after a lifetime of exposure to the high levels of allergens. Well, that year, Helen's hay fever reached a point that she was put on prescription medications for her allergies. The

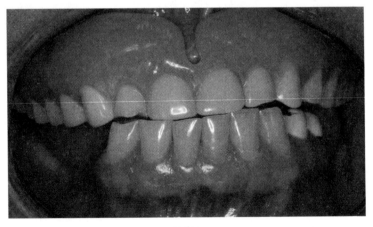

Helen

combination of these medications resulted in her experiencing a severe dry mouth, which she then self-treated with lozenges, Life Savers, and cough drops. By the time Helen made it to her next checkup appointment, she had twenty-two new cavities. As I attempted to figure out what had gone wrong and explain to her what I believed was happening, she grew frustrated and left my office. She transferred to another dentist, and I didn't see Helen again for six years. Sadly, when she finally came back to my practice, she had only eight remaining teeth. She apologized for not believing me and listening to my advice. I am sorry that I wasn't able to help her. What was once a beautiful smile had been reduced to rubble by this disease. What exactly went wrong? Read on to get the full picture.

Have you ever noticed that some people do everything their dentist recommends yet still get cavities whereas some don't seem to care about their teeth at all and have never experienced the drill? It seems so unfair! One of the main reasons we think cavities seem to show up when they shouldn't—or don't show up when they should—is our limited understanding of how and why we get cavities. For starters, most people don't know that cavities are caused by a malfunction in your biofilm. Biofilm is a scientific term for a thin, sticky layer of bacteria and microbes. All people have a biofilm on their teeth; each biofilm is unique, made up of a complex network of living microbes. The biofilm is not a bad thing; in fact, having a network of healthy bacteria and microbes on your teeth is a good thing! A healthy biofilm actually protects your teeth. Problems arise when environmental factors influence how your biofilm behaves.

Wait, you've lost me . . .

Think of your biofilm as a garden. You want a healthy garden full of yummy vegetables and beautiful flowers. To have a healthy garden, you must influence the growth of good plants. You pull the weeds as they pop up, you apply weed killer, you watch out for pests like slugs and snails, you water and apply fertilizer to the good plants, and so forth. You are using what scientists would call selection pressure—your environmental influence controls which plants survive and which ones die off.

Selection pressure: The extent to which organisms possessing a particular characteristic are either eliminated or favored by environmental demands.

Nerd Alert

Say you go on vacation and while you are gone, your garden is left unattended. The environment and selection pressure have changed (the protector of the good plants and killer of bad plants is gone); what do you think will happen to your garden? Chances are that pests will invade and that when you get home, you will have a weed patch instead of a garden. The same concept can be applied to a biofilm.

Biofilms and gardens? I don't get it!

The biofilm is a network of thousands of different kinds of microbes. Most are good, and some are bad, and for your teeth, some are extremely bad. The selection pressure—or the mechanism that controls whether your biofilm is functioning normally and is healthy or whether it is malfunctioning and causing damage—is pH.

pH is a number between 0 and 14 that indicates if a chemical is an acid or a base. Lemon juice has a pH of about 2.5. Water has a pH of 7, which is neutral.

Nerd Alert

Just like you, the gardener, provide the selection pressure on your garden, controlling which plants live and which get weeded out, pH is the selection pressure for the biofilm on your teeth. As the pH of the mouth changes, the way the biofilm behaves changes too. Specifically, if the pH drops below 5.5 for extended periods, the weeds grow, and the flowers die off. If the pH is kept above 5.5, the reverse is true.

What does biofilm behavior have to do with cavities?

Great question; I'm glad you asked! Through some pretty complex systems, the behavior of the biofilm controls whether minerals are staying in the teeth (healthy) or are moving out of the teeth (decay). If, for example, the pH of your mouth stays below 5.5 for a long period, the biofilm becomes imbalanced, and it begins to eat away at the minerals that make up the teeth. You can see where we are headed with this, right? As minerals are removed from the teeth, holes form in the enamel. Then the microbes invade your teeth, and these holes are what we know as cavities.

In a nutshell

To recap, we all have biofilms on our teeth. A biofilm is a complex network of bacteria and microbes (like a garden full of flowers and weeds). The selection pressure, or environmental variable that controls how this garden behaves, is pH. If the pH is too low, the biofilm becomes sick and begins to eat away at the enamel, causing cavities. Whew!

pH below 5.5 = bad bacteria thrive = cavities
pH above 5.5 = good bacteria = health

Pay Attention

If pH controls the biofilm, what controls the pH?

Ah, and here is where things get really interesting. The pH in your mouth is not static; it is constantly fluctuating throughout the day and night. Just about anything you put in your mouth can have an effect on your oral pH: eating and drinking, lack of saliva, smoking, drug use, medication use, oral appliances, brushing your teeth, or rinsing with mouthwash. If you put something in your mouth, it is going to positively or negatively affect your oral pH. We will learn more about the details throughout the book; for now, understand that pH is dynamic and that it is the underlying factor for everything else we will discuss. Now let's talk about the major influences that help your dental professional determine whether you are at risk for having (or getting) a sick biofilm.

The 5 Factors

Your dental professional should look for five factors when determining what is causing your decay. In my forty years of practice, seeing thousands of patients, the underlying causes of patients' cavities almost always boil down to one or more of these five issues:

1. Lack of saliva
2. Poor diet
3. Imbalance of the biofilm
4. Genetics
5. pH

An experienced dentist or hygienist can figure out the cause of your cavities by asking a series of pretty easy questions. These questions are also known as the Caries Risk Assessment, an important step in P4 Dentistry. It's an excellent predictive tool to help detect a potential problem before it develops into an acute infection.

If you want to sound extremely well informed, ask your dentist if the office has a Caries Risk Management program. This is a fancy industry term for asking patients questions to figure out which of the five factors apply to them. This can help you and your dental care team personalize your treatment plan for maximum oral health.

Each of these five factors will get its own chapter for more depth, but here's a quick breakdown.

1. Lack of saliva or dry mouth

Saliva is important. It is your mouth's natural defense system. It washes contaminants away from your teeth. It helps return your mouth's pH level back to neutral after eating. It bathes your teeth 24/7 in the exact mineral your teeth are made of.

When you don't have enough saliva, your teeth are exposed to a great deal of additional stress. The cavity-causing microbes thrive without the protection of the saliva. This upsurge can cause cavities and bad breath. The high-acid environment that builds after eating does not return to normal due to the lack of saliva, leading to a loss of minerals, which causes a loss of enamel. Dry mouth is a direct risk for your teeth.

What causes dry mouth?

There are several possible reasons for dry mouth. One is the natural aging process. As we grow older, many of our body's systems don't function as well as they did when we were younger. Another common cause is medication use. Dry mouth is a remarkably regular side effect for many of the most common types of prescription and over-the-counter medications.

Several medical conditions can also cause dry mouth. Some, such as Sjögren's syndrome, are genetic. Diabetes is frequently accompanied by dry mouth, as are several other chronic medical conditions. Smoking also can decrease saliva production, as will vaping. We will learn more about dry mouth in Chapter 2.

2. Damaging diet and frequent eating habits

This one is a doozy and probably the most difficult factor to discuss. A person's beliefs about food can give politics and religion a run for their money as a conversation topic. I like to stick to the science and let patients decide for themselves what to take and what to leave behind. What we know is that every time we eat or drink, the pH in our mouth drops. When that happens, the bad microbes in the biofilm feed and create acid waste, resulting in mineral loss in the teeth. If this happens frequently enough or for long enough durations, the biofilm will become sick or imbalanced. Once this happens, it is difficult to correct.

But . . . I am a raw vegan who hasn't had sugar since 1976!

Most dental professionals focus on sugar when talking about diet and cavities with their patients. This isn't wrong, but it is a prime example of how we have oversimplified and thus misinformed the mainstream. Sugars play a role, no doubt about it, but there is far more to the story. We will further unpack diet in Chapter 3. Even if you are a raw vegan who avoids sugar like the plague, read Chapter 3—I promise there will be information that will apply to you.

3. Biofilm

Oral biofilm is much like the ocean floor or outer space; it's so vast that we will be exploring and learning about it for decades to come. While we typically think of bacteria when we use the term biofilm, it's actually a complex community that contains other organisms besides just bacteria. The oral biofilm also includes yeasts and viruses. We commonly refer to these organisms collectively as microbes, so I'll be using that term in the book when I discuss biofilms. Despite how much we have left to learn, we know enough about oral biofilms at this point to be dangerous. There are a few ways to determine whether the biofilm is sick. Cavities themselves are a sign. Some dentists can measure the bacterial activity with a special device to see if the biofilm contains too many bad microbes, putting you at risk. If none of the other five factors apply to you, and you are getting cavities, chances are good you either have too much biofilm on your teeth, you have too many of the wrong kind of microbes in your biofilm, or your biofilm is behaving badly.

4. Genetics

This is an emerging science. We know that genetics plays a role in a person's susceptibility to a biofilm becoming imbalanced—and also in how responsive the biofilm is to treatment—but how much genetics contributes and what genes are involved are still being researched. It is safe to say a person's genetics and interaction with the environment at a basic level are what cause the disease. We will explore genetics in Chapter 5; if none of the other five factors resonate with you, I would make sure to read what we know at this point about genetics and decay.

5. pH

As we discussed earlier, pH is the selection pressure for the way your biofilm behaves. At this point, it is important for you to know that saliva, diet, biofilm, and genetics all influence the pH in your mouth. If you have a diseased biofilm, it is safe to say your oral environment is spending far too much time below the pH of 5.5. The good news is that just as you can influence your pH in the negative, you can also control elevating your pH, which, given enough time and exposure, can alter the biofilm back to health. But I'm getting ahead of myself. We will go into the details later in the book. Stay tuned.

How Does This Apply to Me?

If the cause of my cavities is a sick biofilm and there are five risk factors contributing, do I believe patching the hole cures it?

Ask Yourself

Here's where the rubber meets the road. You are spending a great deal of your hard-earned money filling holes in your teeth with the expectation that it is fixing the problem. Guess what? It's not. Fillings are likely the most misunderstood part of the whole cavity process. Most of my patients have gone to the dentist their whole lives, had cavities, have had them filled, thought the problem was resolved, and then found themselves with another cavity six months later. They do not fully understand that *we could have treated the biofilm imbalance and prevented the second cavity from happening*. How? By changing the environmental elements and possibly introducing an antibacterial treatment. The filling is important—don't get me wrong—but it does not solve the underlying conditions that caused the cavity in the first place. Left uncorrected, cavities will continue to develop. Traditionally we focused on how many cavities patients had rather than figuring out why they had cavities in the first place.

I don't want to sound like a broken record, but that changed for me personally about twenty years ago when I started exploring why patients had cavities to begin with. If you don't know what's causing your cavities, your oral health is turned into something of a game of whack-a-mole, and the consequences are much more serious than cavities alone.

This Is about More Than Your Teeth

Oral infection has been linked to heart disease,[1] Alzheimer's,[2] dementia,[3] stroke,[4] diabetes,[5] among other life-threatening conditions.

Pay Attention

To take care of your teeth is to take care of the rest of your body. Although medical doctors (MD) work in different offices than do doctors of medicine in dentistry (DMD) or doctors of dental surgery (DDS) and have different insurance billing systems, your body is a single unit; so treating the mouth in relation to the rest of the body is the reason cavities are more than just holes in the teeth. They are an imbalance in the body that affects the entire system. It is ridiculous to patch the hole and assume you are cured of the disease. Treatment needs to look at the big picture, which will include taking personalized steps to predict and prevent future disease.

BITE-SIZED TAKEAWAY—**Filling a cavity isn't enough; you also need to look at the circumstances that lead to cavities in the first place!**

Chapter 2

Why Me?
My Mouth Is So Dry!

Ask Yourself

Do I take medications daily?

Does my mouth feel dry at any time during the day or night?

Do I need to keep a glass of water by the bed to drink at night?

Do I chew gum or suck on candy to keep my mouth moist throughout the day?

If you answered YES to any of these questions, this chapter is particularly relevant for you.

IN THIS CHAPTER:

- Saliva—A super tooth keeper.

- Dry mouth is surprisingly common—you are not alone!

- Medicating your way to a higher risk.

- What else can cause dry mouth?

- It can happen to anyone.

Renee is one of my favorite patients. She first came to see me about twenty years ago when she was thirty-five years old. She has a beautiful smile and is a warm, and friendly soul. Renee was frustrated because she believed that she was doing an excellent job of brushing and flossing her teeth, yet she was getting about two new cavities every year as an adult. Her previous dentist told her that she needed to brush and floss better. I looked in her mouth. I have to tell you, I was shocked. She had the best hygiene and the cleanest mouth I had ever seen. Her home care rivaled

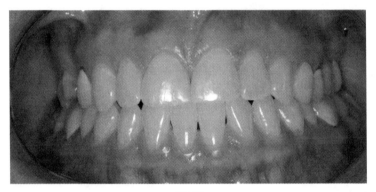

Renee

the best hygienist ever. Clearly her problem was not a biofilm issue; she was doing a commendable job. So I began to investigate her risk factors: saliva, diet, biofilm, and genetics. When I looked at her medical history, I saw that she was taking two medications that notoriously cause severe dry mouth side effects. She confirmed that she struggled with dry mouth symptoms daily. Though she wasn't self-treating the symptoms with sugar-sweetened items, her lack of saliva put her at high risk for cavities. We spent some time talking about management strategies that would help her, and she is decay-free to this day. Too often we professionals just give lip service to the old one-size-fits-all mentality and don't look for the specific risk factors driving each individual's disease. I'm happy to report that that is changing. A new focus on personalized medicine allows patients to benefit from a treatment plan focused on which preventive factors will actually make a difference to their care.

Saliva—Super Multitasker and Tooth Preservative

It's easy to overlook the importance of saliva, but it's hard to understate the importance of saliva to the health of your teeth. Saliva is a hard-working multitasker in your mouth, working with several body systems to maintain health. It works with the digestive system to help digest food. It works with the immune system to help fight off germs of all sorts entering through the mouth. Yet, its most important function in the body may be as an active defense your body employs to keep your teeth mineralized.

Your teeth are, in fact, made up largely of minerals. You probably have heard about the importance of calcium, a mineral, for bone health. You may have even heard about having the right amounts of other minerals, such as magnesium or phosphorous, for bone health. What you may not realize is that your teeth are made up of the same kinds of minerals that build strong bones. And, while your skeleton is not surrounded by an acidic environment, your mouth frequently becomes acidic after you eat. If you ever did the chicken-bone-in-a-glass-of-soda experiment as a kid, you know what acid does to these minerals. Acidic conditions in the mouth can dissolve minerals out of the teeth, making teeth susceptible to caries.[6]

Saliva, then, is tasked with keeping the acid levels down and the mouth's pH level elevated. Saliva also captures and replaces the minerals dissolved out of the tooth enamel during acidic conditions. It is a supersaturated solution of the minerals teeth need, and contains proteins and antibacterial, antiviral, antifungal, and pH-balancing elements.[7] It's been said that without saliva, we wouldn't have teeth.

Nerd Alert

Supersaturated Solution: An unstable solution that has more dissolved material in it than usual. The dissolved particles easily fall out of the solution. In the case of saliva, this means the minerals easily come out and can deposit in tooth enamel.

A Surprisingly Common Occurrence: You Are Not Alone!

For a medical condition that rarely gets discussed seriously, dry mouth is a remarkably common condition. Because saliva protects the teeth, dry mouth is a major risk factor for dental disease.[8] Practically everyone suffers dry mouth at some point, even if just for a short period. Despite that only a small number of people will tell their dentist or doctor that they are experiencing dry mouth, studies have shown that dry mouth affects between 20 and 46 percent of the total population.[9] A recent study even reported it as high as 70 percent in adults who take a prescription medication.

Dry mouth is officially known as xerostomia. Its name is derived from the Greek words xeros meaning "dry" and stoma meaning "mouth".

Nerd Alert

Women tend to suffer from dry mouth more frequently than men.[10] It is more common as we age, being relatively uncommon in young children and middle-aged people. Dry mouth is worse during sleep, as well, because our bodies naturally make less saliva during sleep.

At this point, you may be wondering if you have been ignoring signs of dry mouth that could be dangerous for your teeth. If you're reading this chapter, there's a good chance you're already aware of having dry mouth. If you are still unsure if you should talk to your dentist about your dry mouth, consider the following questions:

Does my mouth feel dry?
Do I notice a lack of saliva in my mouth?
Do I get up at night to drink?
Does my mouth feel dry when I am eating a meal?
Do I have a hard time swallowing certain foods?
Do I need to sip liquids to help swallow foods?

Ask Yourself

Do I suck on sweets or cough drops to relieve my dry mouth?

Does my throat constantly feel dry?

Does my mouth become dry when speaking?

If you find yourself answering yes to any or all of these questions, take the time to talk about your dry mouth with your dental professional at your next visit. It's an important step to participating in your oral health care.

Medicating Your Way to a Higher Cavity Risk

Thousands of medications can cause dry mouth. It's a common side effect of both over-the-counter and prescription medications. And we're taking a lot of medications. Seventy percent of Americans of all ages take at least one prescription medication every day.[11] Some extremely common types of medications can cause dry mouth as a side effect. Pain medications, antidepressants, medications to reduce high blood pressure, acid reflux medications, anti-seizure medications, anti-anxiety medications, allergy medications, and cold medications all carry the risk of causing dry mouth, and that isn't even a full list of all possible medications that can cause dry mouth.

Additionally, the risk of dry mouth increases with each additional medication you take daily. Of people who take one medication every day, between 20 and 30 percent experience significant dry mouth. If you take six or more medications a day, your risk for dry mouth shoots up to 60 percent.[12] Reducing the number of medications you take can reduce your risk of dry mouth and improve your oral health, but because the kinds of medication that cause dry mouth are often life sustaining, you may not be able to reduce risk by ceasing to take a medication. Surveying my own patients over the years, 63 percent of them self-identify symptoms of dry mouth at some time of the day or night. So this is a common problem—and one of the most common of the risk factors for tooth decay.

Therefore, even though you may think that your medications aren't relevant at a dental visit, it's really important to tell your dental team about all medications and supplements you are taking for any reason. Your team needs all the information to participate fully in giving you the best health care possible. If you can't stop a medication that is causing your dry mouth or substitute it for another medication, you can use a combination of saliva substitutes, pH-controlling products, xylitol products, calcium mineral, and extra fluoride to balance out the effects of medication-caused dry mouth.

What Else Could Be Causing My Dry Mouth?

Less than 20 percent of people who are not taking any medications experience dry mouth.[13, 14] Some genetic traits or behaviors you engage in could be causing or aggravating dry mouth. Stress can cause dry mouth. If your parents suffer from dry mouth, it's possible to inherit dry mouth from them—your parents' dry mouth may be a predictive factor for your oral health. As you age, you are more likely to have symptoms of dry mouth. Poor diet can also cause dry mouth. Among the other risks of tobacco use, it can cause dry mouth and reduced saliva.

Mouth breathers often experience dry mouth at night. If you sleep with your mouth open, you may wake up in the middle of the night and feel like your mouth is the Sahara Desert and then need to take a drink of water just to be able to swallow. People with sleep apnea and using a CPAP often experience symptoms of dry mouth.

Some chronic medical conditions often go hand in hand with dry mouth. Diabetics often suffer from dry mouth. This may be related to the medications they need to control their blood sugar, or it may be related to high blood sugar levels. Also, if you need to have radiation to treat head or neck cancer, that lifesaving treatment may damage the glands that make saliva. That can cause lifelong dry mouth. In addition, autoimmune diseases, in which your immune system attacks healthy body tissue, can damage the salivary glands. Sjögren's syndrome is one such disease. It can be tricky to recognize and often leads to long-term dental problems. Predictive medical testing can help you hunt down some of these factors, letting you address dry mouth before it begins causing cavities.

If any of these dry mouth causes are giving you an unhealthy mouth, the treatment is the same as medication-caused dry mouth. A combination of saliva substitutes, pH-balancing products, oral care products with xylitol, calcium mineral, and extra fluoride can help preserve tooth health in the face of dry mouth.

No one likes being awakened early on a weekend morning, but a close relative called me one Sunday morning at about 5:30 am. Charlene and her husband had been patients from the beginning of my practice. They were now retired and spending their winters in Palm Desert. Charlene woke up that morning in a panic, with her face swollen and a throbbing toothache. She was another patient whose teeth I had restored early in my career, and she had been decay-free for twenty-five years. She never missed a checkup and did an excellent job of brushing and flossing. Fortunately, I knew a colleague close by. He was kind enough when I woke him up with my phone call, and he arranged for a specialist friend of his to see Charlene that morning and perform a root canal treatment on the infected tooth. I was a little bit perplexed. She hadn't had any dental issues for years and was doing everything right; I was caught off-guard. When she and her husband returned home that spring, I saw her and completed the restoration of her tooth with a crown. I had the chance to start asking her about saliva, diet, and biofilm. It turns out that she had failed to disclose on her medical history update at our previous checkup that she had been diagnosed with high blood pressure and was now taking two medications every day. She subsequently developed a very dry mouth and was self-treating her symptoms with lemon drops. That information would have been helpful at the time, but fortunately I was able to help her understand her risk factors, and she has been decay-free since then. Does her story sound familiar? As I continue to treat this disease, I see it present in regular patterns. It's pretty simple when you start to understand it.

See the following chart for pH values of some common oral moisturizers.[15] This can help you choose ones that are more effective.

Take Action

PRODUCT	MANUFACTURER	pH VALUE
CTx2 Spray	Oral BioTech, Albany, OR, USA	9.09
Dy Mouth Spray	Thayers Natural Remedies, Westport, CT, USA	6.30
Mouth Kote	Parnell Pharmaceuticals, Inc. San Rafael CA, USA	3.03
Oasis	Oasis Cnsumer Health, Cleveland, OH, USA	6.33
Bioténe Oral Balance	GlaxoSmithKline, Raleigh-Durham, NC, USA	6.61
Bioténe Moisturizing Mouth Spray	GlaxoSmithKline, Raleigh-Durham, NC, USA	6.11
Rain	Xlear Inc. American Fort, UT, USA	7.10
Elmex Erosion Protection	GABA, Therwil, Switzerland	4.0
Flux Dry Mouth Gel	Actavis, Petach Tikva, Israel	5.5
Flux Mouthwash	Actavis, Petach Tikva, Israel	5.2
Gum Hydral Gel	Sunstar, Etoy, Switzerland	5.3
Gum Hydral Rinse	Sunstar, Etoy, Switzerland	5.4
Gum Hydral Spray	Sunstar, Etoy, Switzerland	5.3
HAp+	Ice Medico, Reykjavik, Iceland	3.4
Saliva Orthana	A.S. Pharma, Hampshire, UK	5.8
Xerodent	Actavis, Petach Tikva, Israel	6.1

Source: https://www.ncbi.nlm.nih.gov/pmc/articles/PMC5546593/

BITE-SIZED TAKEAWAY—Medications, diet, tobacco, chronic health conditions, and overall health can cause dry mouth. Treat dry mouth using saliva substitutes with a pH of 7 or higher,[16] pH-balancing restoratives, xylitol, and extra fluoride.

Chapter 3

Why Me?
Diet Diaries

Do I snack (even on healthy foods!) between meals?

Do I drink things other than water?

If you answered YES to any of these questions,

Ask Yourself **this chapter is particularly relevant for you.**

IN THIS CHAPTER:

- Food and drink that lower pH damages teeth, not just sugar

- How the modern American diet has changed

- It isn't always about sugar—frequency matters

- Patient example—runner eating energy gels

Marilyn came to me as a teenager. Her parents had spent thousands of dollars on her teeth, and she continued to get severe cavities. She already had numerous crowns, and there seemed to be no end in sight. To be frank, her teeth were a mess. Her parents had given up hope and felt like they were wasting their money. So they brought Marilyn to me to have a set of dentures made so they could eliminate this tooth nightmare. She was seventeen years old. I looked at her and saw a trembling kid who was confused and scared. I suggested that we call official time-out on the field and try to figure out what was causing her decay to see whether there was some hope for her. But her parents were adamant; they were through wasting good money on bad teeth.

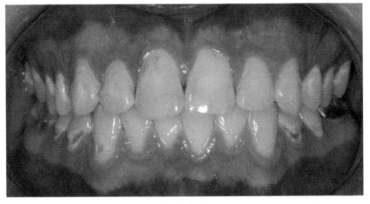

Marilyn

I begged and pleaded and finally got them to agree to let me do a risk assessment, and in return, I agreed that if I couldn't come up with any answers, I would make Marilyn a set of dentures as they had requested. Now my back was against the wall; the last thing I ever wanted to do was subject a seventeen-year-old kid to a lifetime of wearing dentures. I sat down with Marilyn and had a serious meeting of the minds. I told her if she and I didn't figure this out and quickly, she'd be going to her senior prom with a set of dentures. I had a sample set of dentures on my desk and had her hold them to emphasize the point. Then we went through the risk factors—saliva, diet, biofilm, and genetics—together like I always do. She had plenty of saliva. Her diet answers revealed that she was drinking six cans of sugar-sweetened, citrus-flavored soda every day. She also could improve her brushing and flossing, but in my mind the major culprit clearly was the soda. We discussed this at length together and with her parents. I convinced them to agree to let me place some temporary restorations and then let Marilyn work on making the necessary changes for six months to see if we could end this decay cycle. I'm happy to report that Marilyn was successful and went to her senior prom with her own beautiful smile. She has been decay-free since then, and dentures will never be a part of her future. You may know somebody like Marilyn in your own life.

There's So Much More Than Sugar

You want to be healthy, and a balanced diet is likely part of your overall wellness plan. When it comes to eating healthy for your teeth, you've probably been told since you were little that sugar will damage your teeth. That may even be all that you've ever heard about a tooth-healthy diet—avoid sugar and you can keep your teeth healthy. In this model, less candy equals healthy teeth. In surveying my own patients, 55 percent of them self-report that they are eating too much sugar in their diet or that they are eating too frequently.

It turns out that the amount of sugar you eat is only part of the picture. Whenever you eat or drink something other than plain tap water, you change the environment inside your mouth. Your mouth becomes more acidic, or, to put it in more scientific terms, your oral pH level drops.

Nerd Alert

pH level: A standard measurement scale that helps quantify how acidic or basic a substance is. Lower numbers are more acidic, 7 (tap water) is neutral, and higher numbers indicate a base. It is based on how active hydrogen is in the solution.

As you may recall, the pH level of your mouth is important for several reasons. Acidic conditions in your mouth help begin the digestive process; however, they can also dissolve minerals from your tooth enamel. Additionally, the usual pH levels of your mouth help determine the types of bacteria and other microbes that survive best in your particular biofilm. Microbes generally associated with healthy oral environments thrive at higher pH levels. Lower pH levels allow bacteria and microbes that tend to cause cavities to thrive.

In some ways, the pH level of your mouth is like the vibe of a club. Certain pH levels will attract certain types of microbes just as certain vibes will attract certain types of patrons to a club. Your goal is to attract the best and brightest, the most beautiful, to your environment.

How does all this relate to sugar?

In reality, the total amount of sugar you eat is not the main factor that influences which bacteria and microbes are feasting in your mouth. Studies have shown that as these microbes feast on the sugar you've eaten, oral pH levels drop. It's actually the bacteria and microbes metabolizing the sugar that make good players die off and allow less healthy players in the biofilm community take over.[17] The longer the microbes feast, the bigger the negative effect on the oral environment. Again, it comes back to pH.

But I don't eat junk food!

It's not just an added sugar problem. It's not just what you eat; it's how you eat it that counts. Lots of healthy foods are made of nutritional building blocks that your oral bacteria eat for energy. Even eating healthy snacks all day long puts severe strain on your mouth's ability to keep its pH level high and safe. Constantly feeding the biofilm allows too much acidic time in the mouth, which can lead to mineral loss, unhealthy microbe overgrowth, and, finally, cavities. Nibbling, grazing, and sipping all day long prolongs those periods of low pH and helps select for the wrong microbes. It's a lot healthier to eat separate meals and limit snacking. Coffee, even black coffee, may seem like it shouldn't cause a problem. And if you have a cup of coffee or two with a meal, maybe one during a coffee break, it shouldn't be a problem. But coffee itself is already acidic, and you get into trouble when the coffee is sitting on your desk and you sip from it all day long.

It's also worth thinking about those diet sodas you want to believe are safe for your teeth. It's not only sugary beverages that change your oral pH. Any drink other than tap water can lower your oral pH. That's particularly true for carbonated beverages, such as diet soda. The carbonation in soda causes a weak carbolic acid in the beverage, and flavorings can further acidify the drink; whether sugar sweetened or diet soda, both can damage tooth enamel.

Not All Change Is Progress

If we look back over the last fifty to a hundred years, it's undeniable that the way Americans eat has changed. These population-wide changes, unfortunately, have not necessarily been improvements. We eat a great deal more overall, and we tend to eat a lot more of some foods that don't generally benefit our health.

In the last fifty years, our calorie consumption has increased more than 20 percent.[18] We also eat half our calories from grains and fats, a major shift from half a century ago when we ate more fruits, vegetables, meat, and dairy—in other words, whole foods, not processed stuff. We eat more added sweeteners, but they are more likely to be corn sweeteners than ones from sugar cane or beets. If it comes in a bag, box, or a can, read the label. We also drink a great deal more soda or fruit drinks and less milk than previously.[19] It should be no surprise that sugar is the most addictive substance on the planet, and our sugar intake is off the charts. The average American eats seventeen teaspoons of sugar per day.[20] Some they sprinkle on their food; most of it is hidden in the processed foods we routinely eat as part of the Western diet. I'd encourage you at this point to take a break from reading and go to your kitchen and measure out seventeen teaspoons of granulated sugar into a baggie to see what that looks like. I have to tell you, it's shocking, especially when you consider that the World Health Organization recommends our daily intake be about two-thirds of a teaspoon. If you want to see how far off our diet is, measure another baggie out with that and then compare the two. I routinely carry those two baggies in my briefcase now to pass around during my lectures so dental professionals can grasp what that really looks like. On a side note, I wouldn't recommend traveling with baggies and white powder in your briefcase, although it does lead to some interesting conversations with TSA, and I have gotten to meet Max the drug dog.

The increase in starches and sugars is not great news for oral health. These foods provide quick energy for the biofilm microbes that contribute to cavities, and they are likely to contribute to acidic conditions in the mouth, further threatening enamel health. The overall increase in the amount we eat leaves us with acidic conditions in our mouth for longer lengths of time. If nothing else sways us to eat well, perhaps the health of our teeth should.

It's Really about Frequency

Of course, even the healthiest eaters can end up with a mouth full of cavities, even without consuming a gram of sugar. How can this be?

If you eat small frequent meals, you may have a healthy weight, but you might find your teeth suffering for it. Frequent eating interferes with the natural ability of saliva to protect teeth.

Your saliva is designed to raise your oral pH after eating or drinking. As you eat or drink, your oral pH drops. In addition to allowing unhealthy microbes to grow and proliferate, acidic conditions in your mouth can dissolve minerals out of your tooth enamel. When the cycle is working properly, after eating, your saliva has time to raise your oral pH levels back to the safe zone for your tooth enamel. Minerals that have dissolved out of the enamel redeposit back into the enamel, bringing weakened enamel back up to strength. This cycle occurs every time you eat or drink something. The pH in your mouth is a continually changing dynamic.

If your eating and drinking habits do not give your saliva time to do its job, the cycle is broken. Minerals that have dissolved out of your teeth do not get a chance to redeposit, leaving enamel weakened and vulnerable to further bacterial acid attacks.

Frequent eating and drinking also changes which types of microbes thrive in your oral environment. The types of microbes that typically grow in a healthy biofilm die in long-term acidic conditions. In acid environments, the biofilm on your teeth grows more of the microbes that are associated with cavities. A prolonged acidic pH in the mouth greatly increases your risk for cavities.

Comparing pH of Frequent and Infrequent Consumption

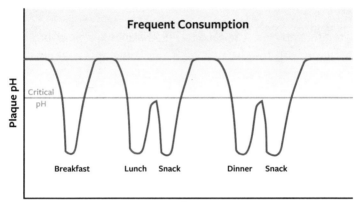

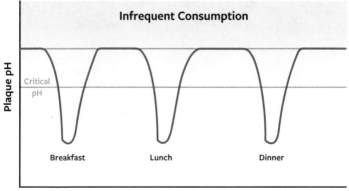

Figure 1: Changes in plaque pH in an individual who (top) has frequent food and drink intake during the day, or (bottom) limits intake to main meals. Teeth demineralize below critical pH of 5.5.

But I need to eat

Sometimes, we just need to eat more frequently. It may be neces-sary for people with diabetes to eat more frequent meals to main-tain good blood sugar control. Pregnant women sometimes need small, frequent meals to maintain optimal health. Sometimes, you may even find that the small meal diet is helping you lose weight, so you're not willing to give up your weight-control prog-ress, particularly if that weight loss is helping you improve your health and control other chronic conditions, such as diabetes or heart disease.

There are steps you can take to help balance out your oral pH levels even with frequent eating. Using a high-pH oral product after eating and drinking can help improve the oral environment. This can help keep cavity-causing microbes from taking over your biofilm. It can help shorten the amount of time acid has to attack the minerals in your tooth enamel. By understanding how frequent eating increases your caries risk, the predictive risk, you can take appropriate preventive steps to control for those risk factors.

Take Action *If you are eating frequent meals, use a high-pH oral care product after each meal or snack to help keep your oral environment in balance and protect your tooth enamel from unnecessary damage.*

A Surprising Cavity-causing Supplement

A few years ago, I had a dentist from a neighboring city refer a patient to me for care. This patient was a forty-five-year-old, well-educated, health-related professional who was extremely health conscious. She had been decay-free for almost all her life until about five years earlier. Since then she had been developing an average of two new cavities per year and some years as many as five! Both she and her dentist were frustrated because they hadn't figured out what was causing her problems. Finally, her dentist referred her to me. When I first met Marci, I was immediately impressed by her overall fitness. When I asked about it, she explained that she had taken up marathon running about five years prior and was now into ultra-marathon running. When I inquired about her training regimen, she told me she often ran about a hundred miles per week, mostly after work. I jokingly asked her if she had heard about automobiles, which elicited a smile and a laugh.

I validated that her training program was indeed beyond normal and then asked about her diet. She explained that she typically ate five packets of energy gels during her workday to carbohydrate load for her after-work training run. When I asked more

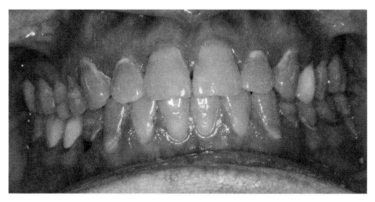

Marci

about that, she explained that she kept the energy gel in her clinic jacket and ate continuously from it during the day until she had consumed five packets. Beyond that, she had a very healthy Mediterranean-style diet, rich in vegetables and fish, and consumed no alcohol. I had never heard of energy gels, but my dental assistant is also a marathon runner, and she happened to have a packet in her car. She retrieved it, and I read the ingredients label. The first three ingredients were sugars with water, followed by essential amino acids and, depending on the flavor, some oil.

So my patient had two issues. She was eating too frequently, not giving her mouth time to recover the pH, and she was eating too much sugar too frequently.

When I explained the process to Marci, and that very likely this one behavior was the cause of her cavities, she asked how she could correct the situation. She decided to eat all five packets at one time right before her daily run and rinse her mouth with tap water immediately afterward. She has been decay-free since then. The energy gel provided her with the energy she needed; it was how she was consuming it that was her problem. Just the change in this one behavior solved her problems. I see similar issues with many patients who are active individuals and misuse sports drinks, foods, and supplements. It's not so much an issue of what these people are eating but rather how they are eating it. But you never find out unless you stop and examine why—until you personalize care.

BITE-SIZED TAKEAWAY—**Diet is one of our modifiable risk factors. We can do better, but making change is really hard. What is one thing you can do today to better your diet?**

Chapter 4

Why Me?
Biofilm (Microbes) Basics

Ask Yourself

Do I notice plaque build-up between brushing?

Do none of the other chapters of this book speak to me, but I am still getting cavities?

If you answered YES to any of these questions, this chapter is particularly relevant for you.

IN THIS CHAPTER:

- ◼ What is a biofilm? Basics on microbes.

- ◼ You may have too many bad microbes or an overload of microbe-causing issues.

- ◼ Acidic microbes deteriorate teeth.

- ◼ How to fight bad microbes.

Bill came to me from out of state. He was in his late thirties and had a disarming smile and laugh. I could tell he had a sense of humor and was a fun person to be around. He had been told that his teeth were not worth saving and that he should think about dentures. By this point you already know where this is going . . . I looked in his mouth and then started with his risk factors: saliva, diet, biofilm, and genetics. It's not rocket science; it's easy. Bill had multiple large cavities, and his teeth were covered in thick discolored plaque. It looked like he hadn't brushed his teeth in ages. He had plenty of saliva and wasn't taking any medications. When we talked about his diet, he shared with me that he drank a few regular sodas during the day. He acknowledged that he could do a better job with his home care. I measured his biofilm with a meter and swab, and it was really high, putting him at risk for more cavities. We discussed the two areas that he needed to modify

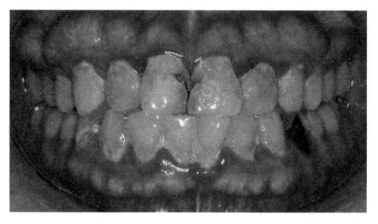

Bill

to get healthy. As a wellness coach, I know that human behavioral change is challenging. Simply put, as humans, we are not good at it. And the one thing I know well is that we're only capable of making one change at a time. So I asked Bill which one he wanted to work on first. I desperately wanted to help him brush his teeth, but he wanted to quit his soda habit. So that's where we started. Six months later, he began working on his brushing and slowly added some flossing to his regimen. In the meantime I restored his teeth; it took several years, but he eventually developed some really good home-care habits. Needless to say, he too has been decay-free since then, and that was almost fifteen years ago. I'll never forget the day he came in for a checkup—I took one look in his mouth, and his teeth were spotless! I spontaneously said, "WOW" in my out-loud voice before I could think, blink, or stop myself. He just beamed and told me he knew I was going to say that. I'm not sure who was prouder that day, he or I.

What Is a Biofilm?

As our understanding of human biology advances, it allows us to grow in our ability to engage in predictive medicine. Growing research helps us better understand the relationship between your health and the millions of little creatures that live in and on your body.

Bacteria are microscopic, living, single-celled organisms that can be helpful or harmful.

Nerd Alert

At its most basic level, a biofilm is a living coating. It is a thin, sticky layer on the teeth that is made up of living things. In the case of your mouth, those living things are mostly bacteria, although there are also yeasts and other microbes. These microbes live, eat, and grow in your mouth, fed by what you eat and drink, growing in the environment set up by your choices and your biology. Whether these microbes in your biofilm are helpful or start making your biofilm sick depends a great deal on what you feed them and the overall environment of your mouth.

OK, but I'm excellent at brushing my teeth.
Can't I just clean it away?

That's not really how biofilm works. Sticky is the name of the game. You can't brush away a biofilm. Moreover, you wouldn't want to if you were to consider the big picture. Much like we now understand that gut bacteria—bacteria that live in your intestine—can be good for your overall health, a healthy biofilm is part of a healthy mouth.

Even if you could brush away your biofilm completely, a new biofilm would quickly begin developing. Don't get me wrong: good oral hygiene, brushing and flossing, is an important part of keeping your biofilm healthy and in check, but it's not the whole story. Not by a long shot. Instead of thinking about how to get rid of your biofilm, it's more productive to consider how to keep your biofilm healthy or how to improve its quality to a healthy, beneficial state. While that could be easier said than done, biofilm can be managed even though it is tricky.

Why is biofilm so tricky?
How is it different from just regular bacteria?

That's something current research is giving us a better picture of all the time. Bacteria in a biofilm act very differently from bacteria that are not in a biofilm. They develop a linked structure that helps them stick together. Once they build up the scaffolding that keeps them together, the bacteria are able to share materials, passing them around. Other microbes in the biofilm act the same way.

Nerd Alert

Biofilms are held together by something called an extracellular matrix. An extracellular matrix is made of molecules that cells excrete to create a structure and support other cells.

They also are able to act together; the bacteria in a biofilm begin to act like a single unit in many ways rather than as a group of individuals.[21] The bacteria act a little like bricks. Picture a bunch of loose bricks spread out in a field; now picture a brick wall. Bacteria can connect with protein strands that act like mortar. The biofilm becomes like a castle wall—connected, strong, and fortified against intruders. Microbes in a biofilm become difficult to penetrate and treat, just like a brick wall.

Though you might be able to fight a group of independent bacteria easily, once they unite into a biofilm, it becomes much harder to influence the bacteria. Think of how much easier it would be to step over a field of scattered stones than it is to get through a fortified stone wall.

Are all biofilms basically the same?

That's not even close to true. All biofilms share certain general characteristics, but they differ considerably in their specifics. Similar to a fingerprint, your biofilm is uniquely yours. But, unlike a fingerprint, your biofilm can change significantly over time—so even your biofilm isn't the same as itself over time.

One of the biggest ways that biofilms can be grouped, how they can vary, is by composition. Biofilm can be made up of mostly one type of bacteria or have a mix of bacteria in it. Another way they can differ is by the overall number of bacteria present. Biofilms that grow unchecked tend to have more individual bacteria living in them over time.

OK, But What Does All This Biology Mean for My Teeth?

Let's bring this discussion back home. If you're having regular cavity issues, you may want to know if your biofilm is the problem. The two biggest issues that cause your oral biofilm to shift from healthy to unhealthy are an overgrowth of microbes and an environment that favors allowing unhealthy microbes to grow and dominate the biofilm. To develop a personalized treatment plan, it's important to identify which biofilm issues are relevant to your specific oral health.

Too many bacteria/microbes

If you notice a buildup in plaque on your teeth or if you regularly feel like your teeth are fuzzy, you are probably noticing the buildup of biofilm on your teeth. Chances are that you are brushing and flossing more to try to dislodge the film. If you are feeling this buildup frequently, you have probably also realized that brushing and flossing alone are not stemming the tide of biofilm growth.

The problem is that once a biofilm has attached, it's almost impossible to remove it mechanically (by scrubbing it away). And, once free-floating bacteria have organized into a biofilm, they can be as much as a thousand times more resistant to antibiotic or antimicrobial treatment.[22]

The Wrong Actors

Of course the sheer number of microbes in your mouth, as important as that number is, does not determine the relative health of your oral biofilm as much as the type of microbes that make up the biofilm do.

A healthy mouth has a neutral to alkaline or elevated pH, and the microbes that live in elevated pH conditions can live on tooth surfaces in relative peace. When you eat, the pH level in your mouth drops. Normally, when your mouth is in balance, your saliva raises your oral pH back up to healthy levels after eating. Some of the microbes even help raise the pH during this part of the cycle. Problems arise when this balance is disrupted.

Cavity-causing microbes thrive in acidic, low-pH conditions.

Pay Attention

If you eat frequently or sip non-water beverages throughout the day, your mouth's natural methods of raising pH back to tooth-safe levels can become overwhelmed. This drags your oral environment further out of balance. This might be a good time to talk about the pH of water sources. Tap water tends to be neutral or right around a pH of 7. Many people now exclusively drink bottled water. The pH values for bottled water vary considerably, with about half of the products having a pH around 4, well into the acid range and at a level that would negatively influence your biofilm and enamel. Make sure you know the pH of the water you drink. Tap water is always a good choice. You see, the microbes that cause cavities don't just thrive in acid environments. They also make acid themselves, causing the mouth to be even more acidic. This allows more acidic-loving microbes to grow, which in turn make more acid. Over time, your entire biofilm can shift to being unhealthy.

What's the danger with acidic microbes?

The acid is particularly dangerous to tooth enamel. The minerals in your tooth enamel are dissolved by acidic conditions. If your mouth stays acidic, the minerals can't redeposit in the enamel. The demineralized enamel is weakened. The weak enamel is both where and how cavities develop. Cavities are a disease caused by a dysfunctional biofilm.

How Do I Fight the Dysfunction?

If you suspect a biofilm imbalance, you should consult your dentist for help. A simple test called a CariScreen can help measure the number of microbes in your biofilm. This can help you and your dentist choose appropriate, evidence-based treatment if you have an overgrowth of disease-causing microbes. This testing process can be part of your preventive care plan, as you can identify a biofilm imbalance before it causes active caries disease.

Because biofilm is so difficult to treat, antimicrobials may be part of your treatment plan, but they probably won't be the only part of your treatment plan. Products that correct your oral pH are another useful arrow in the quiver. Raising your pH level makes the oral environment more unfriendly to cavity-causing microbes. Rearranging your eating habits to allow your mouth's natural defenses to work better should also be part of your treatment plan whenever possible.

If you have a biofilm imbalance, it probably developed over time. So you should not expect it to return to a healthy balance overnight. You and your dental team will need to work together to monitor your oral health over time to restore balance. The important thing to remember is that you have an active role to play here.

BITE-SIZED TAKEAWAY—**Our biofilm is complex! The good news is you can have an effect on how your bacteria grow and affect your risk!**

Chapter 5

Why Me?
Genetic Jackpot or Jack-not

Ask Yourself

Do I have a history of decay?

Does my family have a history of decay?

Do none of the other chapters of this book speak to me, but I still get cavities?

If you answered YES to any of these questions, this chapter is particularly relevant for you.

IN THIS CHAPTER:

- ■ How much of tooth decay is genetic?
- ■ What kinds of genes affects teeth?
  - ☐ Tooth development genes
  - ☐ Saliva production genes
  - ☐ Taste genes
  - ☐ Other genes
- ■ Examples of genetic tooth decay

One of the many things I do in dentistry is keep abreast of the latest research in tooth decay. I attend research meetings, subscribe to scientific journals, and follow the progress of the research. Each year I read and review as many papers on the topic as I can find. A few years ago now, I was catching up on my journal reading when I came across a new study on the genetic influence in tooth decay. The study was large and looked at numerous genes from hundreds of individuals and tried to establish a link between their genes and their decay history. In this particular study, one gene, LYZL2, was determined to be connected with a very specific pattern of decay, in that the individuals with an expression of this gene had cavities only in their lower front teeth, the mandibular incisors. I remember reading this paper and thinking, I don't buy it. If there is one thing we dental professionals know, it's that these are the most protected teeth in the mouth, and they are generally the last teeth to be lost from any cause. So to see a patient who only had cavities in these teeth seemed far-fetched, and I am sure I had never seen anybody like that. Two weeks later, Jennifer was referred to me by a pediatric dentist. She was twelve years old and had cavities only in her lower front teeth. They had been filled and refilled

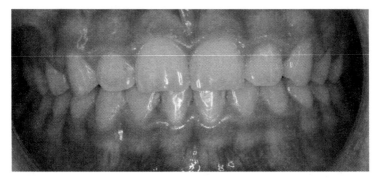

Jennifer

and now needed to be filled again. The pediatric dentist and the mother were very frustrated and came to me to see whether I had any idea of what was going on. I took one look at Jennifer and her X-rays and turned to the mother and explained that it was a genetic condition involving the LYZL2 gene. The mother was stunned that after so many years of frustration, I took one quick look and knew exactly what was happening. I have to admit, I looked like the smartest person in the room for about five minutes. But I'm a truth teller, so I explained to Jennifer's mom that I had only come across this information two weeks prior. And before that, I'm not sure I would have had a clue as to what was causing her unusual pattern of decay.

If you've exhausted all other reasons that you could be suffering tooth decay or feel like there is no answer that explains enough of your caries disease, you might need to look to your family history. P4 medicine stresses the benefits of looking at your genetic risk factors as an important preventive medicine tool.

Your genes may play a role in your tooth decay. Correction— we now know that genes do play a role in tooth decay. For a long time, dentists suspected that genes played a role in tooth disease. Many years ago, dentists told patients that they had "soft teeth." But it wasn't possible until very recently to determine exactly how genetics factored into the process.

Nerd Alert

Genes: The short segments of DNA that tell your body how to assemble proteins and determine which traits you possess.

Genetics: The study of genes and how they are determined in living beings.

Recent advances in genetics and gene mapping, combined with computer analysis, have allowed us to build a better sense of how genes work in everyday health. Scientists have been able to take data from lots of people, examining hundreds of genes and decay experiences, and find patterns. The rapid drop in cost for sequencing (mapping) individual genes has both helped scientists look for these genetic patterns in health and have made discovering genetic risk factors more affordable for individuals.

To What Extent Is My Tooth Health Predetermined?

Based on our current research, and this is a rapidly developing field, it's a pretty good estimate that genes account for around 10 percent of the role in tooth decay whereas environment, social circumstances, and behavior are responsible for about 60 percent or more.[23] It's easy to understand the role played by some of the genes that are now identified with tooth decay whereas others seem to have a more abstract relationship to oral health. Even as you ponder that you may have bad luck out of the gate where your tooth health is concerned, it's important to remember that even if your genes set you up for failure, the environment greatly influences the expression of those genes.

Even if your genes set you up for failure, what you do about them plays a bigger role in your tooth health.

Pay Attention

The remaining percentage of tooth health is associated with professional oral health care. It's frustrating to us, as dental professionals, that there are limits to how much we can help you. The multiple risk factors and complexity of this disease is the reason that tooth decay is the number one disease worldwide, in every country and in every demographic.

The Breakdown: Which Genes Matter?

Tooth development genes

It makes sense that genes controlling tooth and enamel development would play a role in your decay risk. Two genetic conditions are well known to dental professionals to cause poor enamel health and high decay risk. They are *amelogenesis imperfecta* and *dentinogenesis imperfecta*.

Amelogenesis imperfecta causes poorly formed enamel. It is caused by concurrent mutations—mutations that all happen simultaneously—in the AMELX, ENAM, and MMP20 genes.[24] These genes provide instructions for making proteins that are essential for normal tooth development, but the concurrent mutations provide instructions for making defective enamel. These teeth are typically smaller and discolored. They erode and decay fairly quickly after they erupt.

The teeth of a patient with dentinogenesis imperfecta may look similar to amelogenesis imperfecta. Dentinogenesis imperfecta is a genetic disorder of the development of the inner layers of tooth. This condition may be associated with osteogenesis imperfecta, a genetic condition that causes bones to form improperly. Dentino-genesis imperfecta leaves the teeth discolored, translucent, or opalescent. Teeth are weak and can wear quickly, break, and be lost easily. Happily, both amelogenesis imperfecta and dentinogenesis imperfecta are fairly rare, occurring in between one in seven thousand to one in fourteen thousand people in the United States, but not all genetic factors that affect tooth health are rare.

Numerous studies have shown that individual tooth-development genes play a significant role in the average person's decay risk. The AMELX gene, which influences tooth development, has been found in numerous studies[25, 26, 27] to make teeth more suscep-tible to decay if certain mutations are present. Similar evidence has been gathered about the ENAM gene, which governs enamel development. Three genes, AMELX, AQP5, and ESRRB, have supporting evidence, with multiple replications and data, to show that they play an crucial role in tooth decay.[28]

Saliva production genes

Lack of saliva is a major factor in tooth decay. So upon reflection, it is not a huge surprise that genes that influence saliva have been shown to play a role in tooth decay. For example, the AQP5 gene, which we looked at with tooth development, controls a water channel protein, meaning it helps regulate how the body makes saliva.[29]

Saliva is not made of simple water, as you can easily tell. The saliva of healthy individuals contains, among other things, antimicrobial protective enzymes. Beta defensin-1 is an enzyme controlled by the DEFB1 gene that has been studied worldwide because it helps protect the teeth. Saliva also contains minerals that the tooth is made up of. The amount of calcium phosphate constantly bathing the teeth helps keep teeth healthy or makes them more vulnerable to decay. The AMELX, AMNB, and ESRRB genes influence the quality of the saliva by helping control the mineral levels of the saliva solution.[30] Because supersaturated saliva is necessary for teeth, these genes are vital to healthy teeth.

Supersaturated Solution—A solution that contains more dissolved material than usual. Slight disturbances of the solution cause the dissolved materials to form crystals and leave the solution.

Nerd Alert

Taste genes

Taste also plays a major role in tooth decay, mostly because it plays a major role in food choices and eating decisions. We've been able to identify many genes that help regulate taste. For example, the TAS2R38 gene is associated with *supertasters*.[31] Supertasters are extremely sensitive to phenols and other chemicals that are common in cruciferous vegetables. Even though the gene generally loses its expression at midlife, supertasters are prone to eating more sugar because they tend to prefer sweets to vegetables. Obviously, this preference leads to an increased cavity risk. Other genes that influence taste preference for sweets can similarly increase risk factors for tooth decay.[32]

Other unanticipated genetic links

Although we might not have thought of it first, we have found that a change in the human leukocyte antigen DQ2 gene changes decay risk.[33] Upon reflection, it starts to make sense that a change in a leukocyte—a type of white blood cell whose job is to protect our health—would change how well our body can fight off a disease.

While enamel is mostly mineral crystals, the interior of the tooth, the dentin layer, has a large amount of protein present. These proteins hold the living cells of the tooth. Matrix metalloproteinases (MMPs) are enzymes in the dentin, and they assist in the breakdown of protein in dentin. Once we consider that, we can understand the logic behind the role they can play in advancing a cavity inside the tooth. Many of the MMP enzymes—including MMP 2, 13, and 20—are considered factors increasing the risk of decay.[34] Additionally, MMP 20 can increase the risk of dental restoration failure.[35] When we consider why a restoration fails, it's important to consider the possibility that genetics may be partially to blame.

What Does Genetic Decay Look Like in the Wild?

Patients with increased genetic risk generally look just like all other patients. We can now identify some patterns of genetic risk. For example, a patient with a mutation of the LYZL2 gene will end up with decay only in the lower front teeth. The LYZL2 gene influences a protective bacteriolytic enzyme in the saliva. The teeth that are typically the most protected in the mouth and are usually the last to decay are the only ones that show signs of decay when this enzyme protection fails [Figure 2].

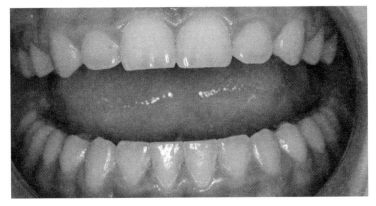

Figure 2: LYZL 2 gene polymorphism. A 14-year-old patient with decay and fillings only in the lower front teeth.

Another pattern that can be identified as a genetic decay pattern is associated with the AJAP1 gene, which influences tooth development.[36] Although people who have a mutation on this gene look like they are developing normal teeth at first, the teeth are not sound and have a significantly increased risk of decay. Despite not having any other clear risk factors for decay, people with this issue will have serious decay very early in life. They may end up with crowns on all their teeth in their teenage years [Figure 3].

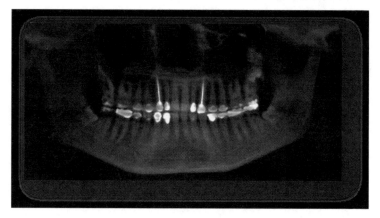

Figure 3: Suspected AJAP1 gene polymorphism, a 14-year-old patient already with 17 crowns and 2 root canals

What can I do? How can I know if it's me?

Unfortunately, aside from a couple of gene variations that create a unique expression and appearance in the mouth, we are not yet able to test your genes to determine whether they are increasing your risk for tooth decay. This is not the end of the story however. Scientists such Dr. David Wong at UCLA are busy working on identifying proteins in the saliva, some of which may be connected to tooth decay.[37]

The world of genetics is rapidly expanding, and we continue to identify more genes that might play a role in tooth decay. At some point in the future, we will be able to use a simple saliva test to check your genetic risks for many diseases, including decay risk. Remember, genes can prep the mouth for certain conditions, but outcomes heavily depend on environmental and behavioral factors. As P4 medicine grows to be the dominant approach in health care and as the cost and accuracy of genetic testing continues to drop, becoming within reach for a majority of patients, our ability to use genetic information to predict and prevent dental disease will grow and improve.

Chapter 6

Why Me?
The pH Phenomenon

Am I a human currently reading a book about cavities?

If you answered YES to this question, this chapter
 Ask Yourself ***is especially for you!***

IN THIS CHAPTER:

- pH affects everyone!

- Basics—Stephan Curve

- pH of dental products, drinks, and bottled water

pH Affects Everyone!

pH levels are a little like blood pressure—everyone has blood pressure that varies a bit throughout the day, but you probably don't think about yours much unless you're having a problem with it. The pH levels in your mouth rise and fall throughout the day, influenced by several factors, between alkaline (basic) levels and acidic levels.

pH: a measurement that tells how many hydrogen ions are in a solution (liquid mixture). It ranges from 1 to 14 and allows us to understand if a solution is acidic or alkaline. pH measurements of 7 are neutral.

Nerd Alert

In addition, just as maintaining a healthy blood pressure helps protect your heart from serious disease processes, maintaining a healthy oral pH helps prevent serious biofilm diseases in your mouth. How does the pH stay steady or change in your mouth, and how does knowing about it help you participate more fully in your health care by controlling your oral pH?

The Basics of Oral pH Changes— the Stephan Curve

Your individual oral pH may be a bit different from that of other people you know, but your oral pH remains steady throughout the day—if you don't eat or drink. As soon as you eat or drink, you start a reaction in your mouth. The bacteria that live in your biofilm begin to feed on the food and drinks you've taken in. The bacteria then excrete acids. This causes the pH level in your mouth to drop, becoming acidic. This process is called a Stephan response.

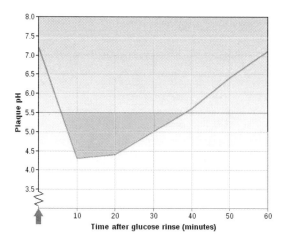

Figure 4: Example of a Stephan Curve showing oral pH dipping and rising after sugar water rinse

When you eat or drink, your oral pH drops quickly. In about five to ten minutes, your oral pH usually bottoms out, becoming as acidic as it will. The saliva in your mouth begins to fight this acid condition, raising your oral pH back up. For most people, this takes about sixty minutes, but it can take longer for others.[38] A Stephan Curve is the curve on a chart, which can be described by a mathematical equation that shows this pH process in action. The charts in Chapter 3 were what occurs with repeated Stephan Curves.

OK, but what does it mean for tooth health?

Your mouth is healthy and happy when it is alkaline. When it is acidic after eating or drinking, the minerals in your tooth enamel dissolve into the saliva, leaving your enamel weakened and susceptible to damage. Your saliva quickly responds by raising the oral pH and giving your teeth a chance to remineralize—take minerals that have dissolved out of the enamel and repair themselves with these same minerals.

If the balance between mineral loss and mineral reincorporation remains through the cycles of pH that accompany eating and drinking, your mouth is healthy. However, if your balance is lost, then you are likely to find yourself suffering from cavities. Long periods of acidic, low-pH conditions cause teeth to lose their minerals without enough recovery time to let the teeth remineralize and restrengthen.

What about the bacteria in my biofilm during acidic conditions?

Great question! The bacteria in your biofilm manufacture acid as a byproduct of sharing in whatever you are eating. Some bacteria and other microbes actually love the acidic conditions and grow better while you are eating frequently or are eating large amounts of the simple sugars that microbes love. Unfortunately, these acid-loving microbes are the same ones that are closely associated with caries disease. They also manufacture more acid to keep the conditions in your mouth just how the microbes like them.

Pay Attention

The more acidic the conditions in your mouth, the more the unhealthy microbes grow, and the more the unhealthy microbes grow, the more the conditions in your mouth stay acidic, favoring the unhealthy microbes.

Biofilm in the mouths of people who eat frequently, regularly triggering low-pH episodes, shifts over time to have more cavity-causing microbes and fewer healthy types of microbes in the mouth. While a healthy mouth with a normal pH balance might have around 113 species of bacteria, a mouth with frequently low pH might only have an average of 94 species.[40]

It's Only Foods That Affect Oral pH, Right?

Nope. Anything you put in your mouth and ingest can potentially alter your oral pH levels. Think about all the things you drink throughout the day. Consider all the oral care products you put in your mouth to help care for your teeth. Everything you put in your mouth can help keep it pH balanced or throw it out of balance.

Wait, did you say oral care products?

That's right. Oral care products can have a huge effect on oral pH, and they are not all created equal. Many are acidic, and some are alkaline. Having an acidic pH in a product may provide for shelf-life stability of the product, but does it make sense to try to reduce acid-loving bacteria by bathing them in acid?

Optimally, your oral care products could utilize an alkaline pH strategy to mimic how nature protects your teeth with saliva. Check with your dentist about which products are safer for your teeth, as information on pH levels in toothpaste can be difficult for the average person to find.

*Well, I don't eat between meals,
but my pH levels are still low. What's happening?*

What are you drinking? Your beverage choices make a huge differ-ence in the pH levels of your mouth. For starters, some drinks bathe your mouth in low pH with each sip, and that's before you consider the additional effect of bacteria using the sugars from those drinks to increase acid conditions. Popular sports drinks tend to have a pH near or under 3, which is extremely acidic. Flavored waters also have a pH near 3. Soda and sugar-sweet-ened beverage mixes, juice, and energy drinks all are listed as erosive dangers for teeth by the ADA.[41]

OK, so I'll skip the flavored drinks for water.

Great! But, while you're doing so, grab a refillable water bottle, and fill it from your tap. Because, as you may be surprised to learn, many commercial bottled waters are acidic. Often, these waters are bottled by soft drink manufacturers and have similar pH to that of many sodas. In addition, as mentioned earlier, acids make it hard for many types of bacteria to grow, so manufac-turers make acidic products to extend the safe shelf life of their products. In fact, some commercial bottled waters have been tested to have a pH level below the level at which enamel starts to demineralize.[42]

It's good practice, not just for the environment, but also for your oral environment, to reuse a bottle filled with simple tap water in most cases. As a bonus, it's probably easier on your wallet as well.

BITE-SIZED TAKEAWAY—**pH is the selection pressure in the disease process. It is constantly in flux and has a huge effect on your biofilm. The good news? You can do things to control it!**

PART TWO:

Taking Action

Chapter 7

Protective Strategies

Ask Yourself

Do I want to know all the available strategies to achieve oral health?

If you answered YES to this question, this chapter is especially for you!

The purpose of this chapter is to provide the resources necessary to make the best choices when choosing your dental products. As covered in previous chapters, we know some risk factors are modifiable (such as diet) while others are not modifiable (such as medications or dry mouth). In addition to knowing your risk factors, it's important to know which ingredients and strategies are best to consider when you're making decisions about dental products.

IN THIS CHAPTER:

- The goal is balance
- pH neutralization by eating less frequently and/or raising pH after eating
- Fluoride
- Xylitol sweetener
- Antibacterial

- Remineralization
- Based on each risk factor—match up appropriate strategies to focus on

I'm always amazed at people's responses to this information. I try to educate all my patients about the best strategies to help prevent decay based on our understanding of the most current scientific research. I vividly recall speaking with an elderly patient who seemed to average about two to three new cavities every year. She was using a commercial toothpaste and mouth rinse and wasn't open to trying something different. My attitude has always been, if those products in fact worked, you shouldn't be sitting here with three new cavities. If it worked, it would have worked. But some people would rather keep doing what they've been doing and continue to get cavities every year. We have many strategies that we can implement to win the battle against decay.

Take Action!

You are not a helpless victim of your oral environment. As we've seen in Part One, cavities are an oral disease and do not happen randomly. There are clear risk factors, and you can take steps to mitigate those risks. Part of being an active participant in your health care is learning all you can so you can make informed health-care decisions, and reading this book can help you with just that. Now that you know which risk factors are most relevant to your specific situation, you can develop a plan based on strategies to counteract your elevated risk factors.

Balance It Out

The human body is full of systems that require balance to function properly. For example, the cardiovascular system requires a careful balance of blood pressure to function properly. If the pressure is too low, blood does not circulate. If the pressure is too high, blood vessels are damaged and wear out prematurely. To keep the circulatory system in balance, you eat right, exercise, control your stress, monitor your progress, and use medications where appropriate.

Your oral health requires a similar balance, as we discussed in Chapter 6. And, just as you can manage your blood pressure, you can take steps to actively maintain the pH balance in your oral environment.

Timing Is Everything

At least when it comes to maintaining a healthy pH, when you eat can be as important as what you eat. Frequent eating and snacking cause your mouth to cycle through low pH too often, overwhelming the saliva's ability to keep pH levels high and healthy. Drinking beverages other than tap water have the same effect on pH levels as frequent snacking does. If you want to maintain a high pH and keep the minerals of your enamel in your enamel, you need to restrict food to regular mealtimes and keep non-water beverages as a mealtime indulgence.

There are some circumstances in which you might not be able to keep mealtimes well spaced-out. If you are a diabetic who requires regular meals or if you have another medical need for frequent eating, you will need to take extra care to support healthy pH levels in your mouth. In these cases, pH-neutralizing oral care products will probably be part of your treatment plan.

If you have identified pH as one of your personal difficulties and are sensitive to damage and shifts toward cavity-causing plaque from prolonged periods of low pH, supporting your oral health with daily high-pH therapy to restore your oral environment to a healthy balance may be beneficial. For preventive purposes, using oral care products with a pH of 8–9 is appropriate. If an unhealthy biofilm has already been established, seek out products with a pH of 9–11 to treat the unhealthy condition. Limited studies performed by the authors of this book have found that wearing trays with a high pH gel at night can have a significant and favorable effect on oral pH and on the composition of the bacteria in the oral biofilm.

Use All the Tools Available

Fluoride is a well-studied tool in the battle against caries disease. It appears to act in several ways: first, strengthening the tooth; second, providing protection against acid attacks; and, third, reducing the amount of acid that cavity-causing bacteria can make.

When the oral environment becomes acidic, the hydroxyapatite that makes up the majority of the tooth enamel's mineral content dissolves out of the enamel surface. If fluoride is present when the hydroxyapatite starts to dissolve, the fluoride combines with the hydroxyapatite to make a new mineral, fluorapatite. When pH rises and the mineral redeposits into the enamel, the new fluorapatite does not dissolve as easily in acid environments, letting the teeth better resist future acid attacks.

You may only think of fluoride in toothpastes or in municipal water supplies as the ways to use fluoride for your teeth, but you have other options to discuss with your dental care team. Your fluoride product recommendations will depend on your Caries Risk Assessment.

The most common fluoride treatment products are:

0.243% neutral sodium fluoride toothpaste/gel (over the counter/ professional)

0.05% neutral sodium fluoride oral rinse (over the counter/ professional)

1.1% neutral sodium fluoride toothpaste/gel (prescription)

5.0% neutral sodium fluoride varnish (prescription)

Young children are susceptible to a condition called fluorosis that can occur if they ingest (eat/swallow) too much fluoride while the teeth are still developing. For children ages two to five, the American Academy of Pediatric Dentistry recommends a pea-sized amount of 0.243% fluoride toothpaste/gel daily. Children younger than two should use a grain-of-rice-sized smear of fluoride toothpaste. Other protective agents, such as pH neutralization, xylitol, and nanohydroxyapatite are appropriate ways to help the youngest children avoid or treat caries disease. For children over the age of six and adults, the appropriate dose of fluoride is determined by the level of caries risk. Your dental care team can help personalize the right set of products that are correct for your particular needs and risk factors.

It's worth noting the scientific evidence clearly favors the use of fluoride as part of your remineralization plan.[45, 46, 47]

Health Can Be Sweet

Xylitol is more than just a sweetener that improves the taste of toothpaste or chewing gum without contributing to tooth decay like refined sugar does. Xylitol is a valuable tool in the fight against cavities in its own right. It is an anticaries agent and makes fluoride more effective.[48, 49] It's worth digging into xylitol to understand why it can be a valuable asset in your fight against caries disease, despite the fact that you may not have been aware of it before reading this book.

Nerd Alert

Sugar alcohols are carbohydrates derived from plants that are poorly absorbed by the body, which means they have a lower impact on blood sugar levels and may cause mild digestive upset. They are called sugar alcohol because part of the molecule resembles sugar molecules, and part resembles alcohol molecules, although they contain neither sugar nor alcohol.

Xylitol is a type of non-nutritive sweetener called a sugar alcohol (although it is neither alcohol nor sugar). It is not often found in over-the-counter dental care products, appearing more frequently in prescription and professional products because it is five to six times more expensive than other more commonly used sweeteners like sorbitol. Additionally, the therapeutic dose of xylitol requires it to be about 10 percent concentration. That means larger amounts of xylitol need to be used than with other non-nutritive sweeteners. Just seeing xylitol on the label is not a guarantee that enough of a dose will be delivered by the oral care product to have a therapeutic effect. It's important to verify the amount of xylitol contained in a product before assuming it will help your fight against dental disease.

Xylitol works to fight cavities in three ways. First, cariogenic bacteria cannot digest xylitol for energy, unlike table sugar and other carbohydrates, so these bacteria cannot use it to produce acid the way that they normally would after you eat. Second, because they do not metabolize xylitol even though they try to, it slows bacteria colony growth and leads to starvation over time. Third, the sweetness of xylitol encourages your mouth to produce more saliva, helping your mouth repair damaged tooth enamel.

When combined with fluoride therapy, xylitol can be even more helpful. Xylitol helps the fluoride be more effective fighting cavities and strengthening enamel. Dental products that combine xylitol and fluoride can be 12 percent more effective in fighting cavities.[50, 51]

Getting Rid of the Bad

If you have an established cavity-causing or cariogenic biofilm, part of your treatment plan will need to include treating the biofilm dysfunction. However, treating a biofilm imbalance is much harder than treating a standard bacterial infection is and poses some additional challenges to eradicating the infection completely.

Free-floating bacteria (planktonic bacteria) are readily treatable with antibiotic therapy. Bacteria in a biofilm are a different matter altogether. Bacteria join together in a biofilm to share resources and protect themselves. As a biofilm grows, it becomes more organized and tightly packed when viewed under a microscope. The more established a biofilm becomes, the harder it is to kill, and the fewer treatment options there are that are effective against the bacteria.[52]

Only three methods exist to completely eliminate an established biofilm. The first is complete mechanical removal, scraping it out and removing it, which is impossible in the mouth. The second way to completely kill a biofilm is to heat it to excess of 400°. Unfortunately, this approach would also kill the teeth along with the bacteria, making it unsuitable for treatment. The third way is to use a broad-spectrum oxidizing antibacterial agent capable of penetrating a biofilm, such as sodium hypochlorite.[53] This, of course, is the method available for dental treatment.

Several antibacterial or antimicrobial treatments have historically been used for the treatment of bacterial biofilms. Ethyl alcohol can be effective, but it also has been linked to oral cancer. Essential oils have been helpful in the treatment of gum infections, but they don't have a body of evidence supporting their effectiveness against cavities. Chlorhexidine has been helpful in fighting plaque caused by *Mutans streptococci*, but it can allow *Lactobacillus* to overgrow and increase as the *Mutans streptococci* is eliminated. Povidone-iodine kills a wide range of germs (bacteria, fungi, mycobacteria, viruses, and protozoans) on contact. It works against *MS* and *Lactobacillus* in children though studies in adults have shown no anti-cavity benefit. It has an unpleasant taste in rinses, and it can only be used once a month to prevent overexposure to iodine. It cannot be used by people with iodine or shellfish allergies. It also stains clothing and surfaces.

Sodium hypochlorite, then, is the preferred option.[54] It is approved for use on patients age six and up, and it may cause an alteration in taste. Because it is a strong treatment agent, it's important to check with your dentist to make certain that you have a bacterial biofilm that would benefit from sodium hypochlorite rinse therapy before adding it to your treatment program. Home use of sodium hypochlorite rinse also can benefit people treating gum disease or canker sores and patients having dental treatment such as root canals, implants, bridgework, and orthodontic treatment.

Firm It Up

In a healthy mouth, the pH cycles of the mouth that naturally follow eating and drinking cause balanced periods of demineralization and remineralization with no mineral loss from the teeth. Minerals lost during low pH return to the teeth when the oral environment cycles back to high pH. If you have caries disease, your balance is lost, and long periods of low-pH, acidic conditions have led to mineral loss. Treating caries disease will involve treating this mineral loss to return your mouth to good health.

Amelogenesis is the process during which tooth enamel develops and covers the inner tooth dentin, which has already grown.

Nerd Alert

The tooth enamel surface is basically a crystal. The crystal surface grows during a process called amelogenesis, during which nanoparticles of minerals floating in a fluid are attracted to larger crystals and attach themselves to the existing crystal structures in an orderly fashion. When your teeth remineralize, hydroxyapatite and fluorapatite attach to the mineral surface the same way that minerals attached during original tooth surface development. For this to happen, the pH level of your mouth needs to be high enough, at least 5.5 for hydroxyapatite and 4.5 for fluorapatite.

The fluid in which minerals float in your mouth (and which makes remineralization possible) is saliva. Several forms of calcium can be found floating in healthy saliva, but they require higher pH levels to begin to attach to your tooth enamel. It is easier for your tooth enamel to incorporate hydroxyapatite and fluorapatite—they have higher bioavailability. Nanoparticles of those minerals (the size the body uses in initial enamel formation) are helpful in replacing minerals lost from your tooth enamel and preventing cavities from developing.[55] Nanohydroxyapatite also can help after tooth whitening by decreasing sensitivity and restoring natural shine to your enamel.[56]

Bringing It All Together

There are things you can do to reduce your risk of developing caries, and there are steps you can take to treat caries disease if you suffer from it. You can weigh your personal risk factors, using current information that is predictive of your risk factors to determine which preventive measures will provide the most benefits to your oral health. Talk over your risks and mitigating treatments with your dental care professional team to build a personal treatment plan to be sure you are taking the best steps possible to maximize your oral health.

BITE-SIZED TAKEAWAY— **You can influence your risk; use as many of these as you can!**

Chapter 8

What's My Plan?

We are going to figure out what, if anything, you would like to do about your risk. I am going to ask you a few questions for you to answer truthfully. Based on where you want to start, come up with an actionable plan, using the modern P4 model of health care, to begin lowering your risk.

1. What risk factor would you like to focus on changing first? If you have multiple risk factors, just pick the one you want to work on first.

_____

_____

_____

_____

_____

_____

_____

_____

2. How has this affected your life?

_____

_____

_____

_____

_____

_____

_____

3. Your options for protective strategies include the following:

_____

_____

_____

_____

_____

_____

_____

4. What do you think you should do?

_____

_____

_____

_____

_____

_____

_____

5. What obstacles might you encounter?

_____

_____

_____

_____

_____

_____

_____

6. How can you overcome or bypass those obstacles?

_____

_____

_____

_____

_____

_____

_____

7. What's the first step toward making this happen? Where do you start?

_____

_____

_____

_____

_____

_____

_____

_____

8. How can your dental professional help you reach your goal?

_____

_____

_____

_____

_____

_____

_____

Action Plan

I **want to** [insert what you want to change] _____

_____

_____ .

because it has negatively affected my life by [insert answer from above] _____

_____

_____ .

I **plan to** [insert answer from above] _____

_____ .

I am going to ask my dental professional to help me with [insert answer from above] _____

_____

_____ .

Chapter 9

Whole-Body Health

IN THIS CHAPTER:

- Your oral health is tied to the health and function of other bodily health

- Heart/Circulatory Health

- Alzheimer's Risk

- Cancer Risk

- Diabetes Management

- Healthy Pregnancy

As I reflect on my career as a dentist, I have so many memories of people whose lives I was blessed to touch. One of the sadder stories involves a patient who had severe gum disease. I have been using lasers for about thirty years and have always done most of my own treatments for gum disease. The laser is an established tool as an alternative technology to scalpels to treat gum disease. I had been encouraging Fred to have his gum disease treated for years, but he always declined treatment. His gums bled, but they had always bled, and he wasn't in any pain. He wasn't concerned. We have known for more than twenty years now that there is some established link between gum disease and heart attacks and strokes. Now we know that one gum-disease-causing bacteria is causal in heart disease. It's not just about your teeth anymore.

Every time I read a new published study on the topic, I shared it with Fred and encouraged him to get his gum disease treated. This went on for many years as I slowly watched his disease progress and progress to the point at which I was concerned his condition was beyond repair and that he was at risk of losing all of his teeth. I'm not sure what I finally said that pushed him over the line, but he finally scheduled for me to begin a laser surgical procedure to treat his disease. Monday morning rolled around and he failed to show for his appointment. We called his home to learn that he had died over the weekend of a massive heart attack. He was forty-eight years old, and he didn't smoke or have any other risk factors for heart disease. I was devastated. I'm not sure that his gum disease caused his death, per se, but it certainly was a risk factor that contributed to it. I will always wonder how this story might have turned out if only Fred had let me treat his gum disease years earlier. We're now beginning to see studies that indicate there may be a risk between some cavity-causing bacteria and other systemic conditions.

The Bigger Picture

Your oral health is not a stand-alone system; it's a part of your overall body health. If you have an oral bacterial imbalance, the effects of that infection are not limited to your mouth. Likewise, health concerns in other parts of your body can complicate your oral care needs. In fact, for certain conditions, dental professionals can often identify areas of concern before symptoms are visible throughout the body. Regular dental care can help with preventive medicine for the whole body. Preserving your oral health is not just important to preserve your teeth; it's also an important step to preserve your bodily health. Let's look at some of the conditions that have been found to be notably affected by your oral health or vice versa.

The Heart of the Matter

The biggest system of the body that poor oral health can damage is the circulatory system and your cardiac health. Periodontitis caused by certain high-risk bacteria has been shown to more than double the risk of heart attack and triple the risk of stroke, conditions caused by a lack of blood flow (circulation), either to the heart in the case of a heart attack or to the brain in the case of a stroke.[57]

High risk bacteria that are found in gum infections, particularly the bacteria *Aggregatibacter actinomycetemcomitans (Aa) and Porphyromonas gingivalis (Pg)*, enter the bloodstream directly from the mouth. This can cause widespread inflammation, a culprit in the worsening of many chronic illnesses. When the inflammation irritates arterial plaques, you can develop blood clots, and a heart attack or stroke generally follows.

After looking at the available materials written about heart and gum disease, the American Heart Association stated that periodontal disease was associated with arteriosclerotic vascular disease. Further study and research have indicated that periodontal (gum) infections from high-risk bacteria are a contributing cause of arterial disease.[58]

You might rightly ask, "*How* much does treating my gum disease matter?" When the doctors studying the relationship between high-risk bacteria and heart disease had the participants in the study manage gum infections, the patients the doctors tracked over two years had measurably improved cardiovascular health, and none of the study participants had a heart attack or stroke during the study.[59]

Reducing inflammation from all sources, including inflammation from oral bacteria and infections, is important in protecting your heart and blood vessel health. Antibacterial treatment is not just tooth and gum sparing; it can be heart sparing as well.

Feeling Foggy?

You may be surprised to hear that your brain's continued functioning benefits from good oral health as well. The increased risk of stroke is not the only threat to your brain from having gum disease. In fact, a study that looked at a group of adults over fifty found a 70 percent higher risk for developing Alzheimer's disease in adults who had gum disease for more than ten years.[60]

It is believed that the inflammation caused by long-term infections, even low levels of inflammation, can damage the brain over time. Patients who have both Alzheimer's disease and periodontitis also show faster decline than those without chronic gum disease.[61]

The Big C

Most of us worry that we or someone we know will contract cancer over the course of our lives. You may be surprised to learn that the inflammation from unhealthy oral bacteria invading the rest of the body increases your risk of developing several types of cancer. You might expect gum disease to increase your risk of head, neck, and oral cancers, and it does. But there are several other cancers that occur more frequently in people with gum disease.

Women with periodontal disease can experience an increase in the rate of breast cancer; smoking further increases the rate of breast cancer in women with periodontal disease.[62] Smoking, of course, also increases the risk of developing periodontal disease to begin with. Pancreatic cancer also occurs more frequently in people who have high levels of antibodies to common periodontal bacteria that have spread throughout the body.[63] Inflammation caused by untreated gum disease is dangerous to healthy cell growth and development and increases your risk of developing cancer. A recent study even implicated another type of oral bacteria, *F. nucleatum*, as a facilitator of colon cancer, making it more severe.

The Sugar Saturation

Diabetes management is made more complicated by periodontal disease. High blood sugar makes diabetics more susceptible to periodontal disease, and gum disease makes it harder to control blood sugar.[64] Diabetes may be noticed by your dentist before you notice it from other symptoms. Uncontrolled blood sugar makes the gum tissue more fragile, bleeding more easily and pulling away from the bone as well as having a distinctive, shiny appearance.[65]

Treating your diabetes and keeping your blood sugar under control is important to help preserve the health of your teeth and gums. Keeping your gums healthy is important because diabetes makes healing more difficult. Diabetes is a body-wide disease, and it requires a body-wide treatment approach to maintain optimum health, which includes taking appropriate steps to protect your oral health.

And Baby Makes Three

Oral care is important in pregnancy, and the more pregnancy dental health is studied, the more we understand how vital it is to the health of mom and baby.[66] Pregnancy complicates oral care. The increased blood flow and hormones that accompany pregnancy can make it harder to keep gums healthy. They are more susceptible to bleeding. Hormones can also cause a benign condition commonly called pregnancy tumors, swollen lumps of tissue that generally go away after the pregnancy is over. The gums are also more susceptible to infections.

Research shows a connection between gum disease and pregnancy issues.[67] Gum disease in pregnancy is associated with premature birth and low birth weight. High levels of cavity-causing bacteria in the mother also are associated with high levels of cavity-causing bacteria in the baby. Taking care of your oral health during pregnancy is an important way to safeguard not only your health but also your growing baby's health.

Balance on the Whole

Instead of delaying dental care or dismissing concerns because they're "just teeth," remember that your mouth is connected to your body and that good health isn't good health if it's limited to just a part of your whole person. Achieving balance in your oral health is an important step toward achieving balance in your overall health.

BITE-SIZED TAKEAWAY— **Gum disease can affect heart health, Alzheimer's, cancer, diabetes, and pregnancy. Taking care of your teeth is taking care of your whole self!**

Chapter 10

Conclusion

Why Me?

We started this journey into your oral health with a question—*why me?* This is a good starting place, but you may have found the answer surprising, taking you to some places you didn't expect when you asked the question. All in all, we find that although you ask what seems like a simple question, the answer can be quite complex. Previously, you may have thought one response—drilling holes and filling them with hard, durable, tooth-replacement materials—was the only way to address cavities. While it's still important to restore teeth to make them biomechanically sound, it's only part of the solution. After reading this book, you should now understand why this is an inadequate response that doesn't address the root of the problem—why the cavity developed in the first place. Caries disease is not simple and straightforward, and treating this disease may require a similarly multistep approach. Examining oral health through the P4 model, focusing on predictive, preventive, participatory, and personalized medicine, can help provide a way to think about caring for oral health in a productive, structured way.

The good news is that this multistep approach is entirely possible. Recognizing all your possible risk factors (predictive) allows you to take corrective steps to reduce or eliminate those risk factors (preventive). Knowing the variety of corrective and protective agents available to you in your fight against caries disease allows you to choose those that will best help you (personalized). Working together with your dental care team (participatory), you can develop a plan to address the heart of the matter—the reasons you have actually developed cavities.

Once you recognize that your oral health is part of your overall health, your goal in treating the caries infection can be part of your whole-person quest for wellness. A healthy oral environment is necessary to avoid inflammation from your mouth spreading throughout your body. You can treat your dental infection with an eye toward reducing or eliminating cavities and gum disease with the real goal of reducing your heart attack and stroke risk factors. Your oral health is intertwined with overall health, and it's important to recognize that the benefits of good health are not limited to just more comfortable dental visits.

As you make your way through this book, you probably found parts that spoke to you directly, parts you really recognized as factors that apply to your life. Take what you learned here and make changes to make your health better. Don't let your enthusiasm end when you shut the book. Enjoy a whole life of better health by taking simple steps and making simple changes that will allow you to look forward to a future that is cavity-free.

And if you know or meet others who are suffering from chronic cavities, please share this book with them. My dream is a whole world of people living cavity-free!

Dr. V. Kim Kutch, DMD

References

[1] https://forsyth.org/news-press-room/connection-between-mouth-bacteria-and-inflammation-heart-disease#.WudJLi7waUk

[2] Shoemark DK, Allen SJ, "The Microbiome and Disease: Reviewing the Links between the Oral Microbiome, Aging, and Alzheimer's Disease," *Journal of Alzheimer's Disease*, vol. 43, no. 3, pp. 725–738, 2015

[3] https://www.europsy-journal.com/article/S0924-9338(11)00124-6/abstract

[4] https://www.sciencedaily.com/releases/2016/02/160216181715.htm

[5] http://www.diabetes.org/living-with-diabetes/treatment-and-care/oral-health-and-hygiene/diabetes-and-oral-health.html

[6] Sreebny LM, Vissink A., *Dry Mouth, the Malevolent Symptom* (Hoboken, NJ: Wiley-Blackwell, 2010), 12, fig. 1.2.2.

[7] Fejerskov O., Kidd E., *Dental Caries: The Disease and Its Clinical Management* (Oxford, UK: Blackwell Munksgaard, 2003).

[8] Domejean S., White JM, Featherstone JDB, "Validation of the CDA CAMBRA Caries Risk Assessment —A Six-Year Retrospective Study," *J Calif Dent Assoc* 39, no. 10 (2011): 709–15.

[9] Sreebny LM, Vissink A., *Dry Mouth, the Malevolent Symptom* (Hoboken, NJ: Wiley-Blackwell, 2010), 12, fig. 1.2.2.

[10] https://www.ncbi.nlm.nih.gov/pmc/articles/PMC4209628/

[11] https://newsnetwork.mayoclinic.org/discussion/nearly-7-in-10-americans-take-prescription-drugs-mayo-clinic-olmsted-medical-center-find/

[12] Sreebny LM, Vissink A., *Dry Mouth, the Malevolent Symptom* (Hoboken, NJ: Wiley-Blackwell, 2010), 92.

[13] Nederfors S., "Xerostomia: Prevalence and Pharmacotherapy, with Special Reference to Beta-adrenreceptor Antagonists," *Swed Dent J* 116, Suppl (1996): 1–70.

[14] Sreebny LM, Valdini A., Yu A., "Xerostomia. Part II: Relationship to Nonoral Symptoms, Drugs and Diseases," *Oral Surg Oral Med Oral Pathol* 68 (1989): 419–427.

[15] Delgado AJ, Olafsson VG, Donovan T., "pH and Erosive Potential of Commonly Used Oral Moisturizers." *J Prosthodont.* 2015 Jul 27. doi: 10.1111/jopr.12324

[16] Delgado AJ, Olafsson VG, "Acidic oral moisturizers with pH below 6.7 may be harmful to teeth depending on formulation: a short report." *Clin Cosmet Investig Dent.* 2017; 9: 81–83. Aug. 3, 2017. doi: 10.2147/CCIDE.S140254.

[17] Marsh PD, "Dental Plaque as a Biofilm and a Microbial Community—Implications for Health and Disease," *BMC Oral Health* 6, Suppl. 1 (2006): S14.

[18] DeSilver D., "What's on Your Table? How America's Diet Has Changed over the Decades." *Pew Research Center,* Pew Research Center, 13 Dec. 2016, www.pewresearch.org/fact-tank/2016/12/13/whats-on-your-table-how-americas-diet-has-changed-over-the-decades/

[19] Gunnars K., "11 Graphs That Show Everything That Is Wrong With the Modern Diet." *Healthline*, Healthline Media, 8 June 2017, www.healthline.com/nutrition/11-graphs-that-show-what-is-wrong-with-modern-diet#section2

[20] http://sugarscience.ucsf.edu/the-growing-concern-of-overconsumption.html#.XMco5TBKiUk

[21] Donlan RM, "Biofilms: Microbial Life on Surfaces." *Advances in Pediatrics.*, U.S. National Library of Medicine, Sept. 2002, www.ncbi.nlm.nih.gov/pmc/articles/PMC2732559/.

[22] Stewart PS, Costerton JW (July 2001). "Antibiotic resistance of bacteria in biofilms". *Lancet.* 358 (9276): 135–8. doi:10.1016/S0140-6736(01)05321-1. PMID 11463434.

[23] Boynes SG, Novy BB, Peltier C., "Risk based treatment planning," *Decisions in Dentistry* February 2017. 3(2):53–57

[24] Smith CE, Poulter JA, Antanaviciute A., Kirkham J., Brookes SJ, et al. "Amelogenesis Imperfecta; Genes, Proteins, and Pathways," *Front Physiol.* 2017; 8: 435.

[25] Kang SW, Yoon I., Lee HW, Cho J., "Association between AMELX polymorphisms and dental caries in Koreans." *Oral Dis.* 2011;17(4):399–406. doi: 10.1111/j.1601-0825.2010.01766.x.

[26] Deeley K., Letra A., Rose EK, Brandon CA, Resick JM, Marazita ML, Vieira AR, "Possible association of amelogenin to high caries experience in a Guatemalan-Mayan population," *Caries Res.* 2008;42(1):8–13. doi: 10.1159/000111744.

[27] Wang Q., Jia P., Cuenco KT, Feingold E., Marazita ML, et al, "Multi-Dimensional Prioritization of Dental Caries Candidate Genes and Its Enriched Dense Network Modules," *PLoS One.* 2013; 8(10): e76666.

[28] Piekoszewska-Ziętek P., Turska-Szybka A. Olczak-Kowalczyk D. "Single Nucleotide Polymorphism in the Aetiology of Caries: Systematic Literature Review." *Caries Res.* 2017;51(4):425–435.

[29] Matsuzaki T., Susa T., Shimizu K., Sawai N., Suzuki T., et al. "Function of the Membrane Water Channel Aquaporin-5 in the Salivary Gland." *Acta Histochem Cytochem.* 2012 Oct 31; 45(5): 251–259

[30] Küchler EC, Pecharki GD, Castro ML, Ramos J., Barbosa F. Jr, et al. "Genes Involved in the Enamel Development Are Associated with Calcium and Phosphorus Level in Saliva." *Caries Res.* 2017;51(3):225–230.

[31] Wendell S., Wang X., Brown M., Cooper ME et al. "Taste genes associated with dental caries." *JDR* November 2010. 89(11):1198-1202.

[32] Ashi H., Lara-Capi C., Campus G., Klingberg G., Lingström P. "Sweet Taste Perception and Dental Caries in 13- to 15-Year-Olds: A Multicenter Cross-Sectional Study." *Caries Res.* 2017;51(4):443–450.

[33] Valarini N., Maciel SM, Moura SK, Poli-Frederico RC. "Association of Dental Caries with HLA Class II Allele in Brazilian Adolescents." *Caries Res.* 2012;46(6):53–5.

[34] Tannure PN, Küchler EC, Falagan-Lotsch P., et al. "MMP13 polymorphism decreases risk for dental caries." *Caries Res.* 2012;46(4):401–7.

[35] Vieira AR, Silva MB, Souza KKA, Filho AVA, Rosenblatt A., et al. "A Pragmatic Study Shows Failure of Dental Composite Fillings Is Genetically Determined: A Contribution to the Discussion on Dental Amalgams." *Front Med* (Lausanne). Nov. 6, 2017;4:186. doi: 10.3389/ fmed.2017.00186. eCollection 2017.

[36] Wang Q., Jia P., Cuenco KT, Zeng Z., Feingold E., et al. "Association Signals Unveiled by a Comprehensive Gene Set Enrichment Analysis of Dental Caries Genome-Wide Association Studies." *PLoS One*. 2013; 8(8): e72653.

[37] https://www.dentistry.ucla.edu/newsletter/18/07/searching-cure-dr-david-wong

[38] The Stephan Curve | Caries Process and Prevention Strategies: The Environment | CE Course. (n.d.). Retrieved from https://www. dentalcare.com/en-us/professional-education/ce-courses/ce371/the-stephan-curve

[39] https://commons.wikimedia.org/wiki/File:Stephan_curve.png

[40] Li Y., Ge Y., Saxena D., Caufield PW, "Genetic Profiling of the Oral Microbia Associated with Severe Early-Childhood Caries," *J Clin Micro* 45, no. 1 (2007): 81–87.

[41] https://www.ada.org/en/~/media/ADA/Public%20Programs/Files/ JADA_The%20pH%20of%20beverages%20in%20the%20United%20 States

[42] http://jdh.adha.org/content/89/suppl_2/6/tab-figures-data

[43] Topping G., Assaf A., "Strong Evidence That Daily Use of Fluoride Toothpaste Prevents Caries," *Evid Based Dent* 6, no. 2 (2005): 32.

[44] American Academy of Pediatric Dentistry Council on Clinical Affairs, "Guideline on Infant Oral Health Care," *AAPD Reference Manual* 33 (2011): 6–11 / 12

[45] Ten Cate JM, Featherstone JD, "Mechanistic Aspects of the Interactions between Fluoride and Dental Enamel," *Crit Rev Oral Biol Med* 2, no. 3 (1991): 283–296

[46] Featherstone JD, Glena R., Shariati M., Shields CP, "Dependence of In Vitro Demineralization of Apatite and Remineralization of Dental Enamel on Fluoride Concentration," *J Dent Res* 69 (1990): 620–625.

[47] Dasanayake A., Caufield PW, "At-Home or In-Office Fluoride Application Does Not Significantly Reduce Subsequent Caries-Related Procedures in Ambulatory Adults of Any Caries-Risk Level," *J Evid Base Dent Practice* 7 (2007): 155–157

[48] Maehara H., Iwami Y., Mayanagi H., Takahashi N., "Synergistic Inhibition by Combination of Fluoride and Xylitol on Glycolysis by *Mutans streptococci* and Its Biochemical Mechanism," *Caries Res* 39, no. 6 (2005): 521–528.

[49] McClendon JF, Foster CW, Ludwick, Criswell JC, "Delay of Dental Caries by Fluorine," J Dent Res 21, no. 2 (April 1942): 139–143.

[50] Sintes JL, Escalante C., Stewart B., et al., "Enhanced Anticaries Efficacy of a 0.243% Sodium Fluoride / 10% Xylitol / Silica Dentifrice: 3 Year Clinical Results," *Am J Dent* 8, no. 5 (1995): 231–5.

[51] Sintes JL, Elias-Boneta A., Stewart B., et al., "Anticaries Efficacy of a Sodium Monofluorophosphate Dentifrice Containing Xylitol in a Dicalcium Phosphate Dihydrate Base: A 30 Month Caries Clinical Study in Costa Rica," *Am J Dent* 15, no. 4 (2002): 215–219.

[52] Cho H., Jönsson H., Campbell K., Melke P., Williams JW, Jedynak B., et al., "http://www.agd.org/ public/ OralHealth/ drymouth/ Dry_Mouth_Brochure.pdf," *PLoS Biology* 5, no. 11 (2007): e302 EP.

[53] http://www.biofilm.montana.edu/

[54] https://www.ncbi.nlm.nih.gov/pubmed/23017003

[55] Allaker RP, "The Use of Nanoparticles to Control Oral Biofilm Formation," *J Dent Res* 89, no. 11 (2010): 1175–1186.

[56] Huang SB, Gao SS, Yu HY, "Effect of Nano-hydroxyapatite Concentration on Remineralization of Initial Enamel Lesion In Vitro," *Biomed Mater* 4, no. 3 (2009): 034104.

[57] Shi Q., Zhang B., Huo N., Cai C., Liu H., Xu J. (2019). *Association between Myocardial Infarction and Periodontitis: A Meta-Analysis of Case-Control Studies.* [online] PubMed. https://www.ncbi.nlm.nih.gov/pmc/articles/PMC5095113/ [Accessed 27 Feb. 2019].

[58] Bale BF, Doneen AL, Vigerust DJ, "High-risk periodontal pathogens contribute to the pathogenesis of atherosclerosis," *Postgraduate Medical Journal* 2017;93:215–220.

59 Cheng H. et al., 2016. "Effect of comprehensive cardiovascular disease risk management on longitudinal changes in carotid artery intima-media thickness in a community-based prevention clinic." https://www.ncbi.nlm.nih.gov/pmc/articles/PMC4947619/

60 Chang C., Wu T., Chang Y., (2017). Association between chronic periodontitis and the risk of Alzheimer's disease: A retrospective, population-based, matched-cohort study. https://alzres.biomedcentral.com/articles/10.1186/s13195-017-0282-6

61 Ide M., Harris M., Stevens A., Sussams R., Hopkins V., Culliford D., . . . Holmes C. (n.d.), "Periodontitis and Cognitive Decline in Alzheimer's Disease." https://journals.plos.org/plosone/article?id=10.1371/journal.pone.0151081

62 Freudenheim J., Genco R., LaMonte M., Millen A., Hovey K., Mai X., Nwizu N., Andrews C., Wactawski-Wende J. (2019). *Periodontal Disease and Breast Cancer: Prospective Cohort Study of Postmenopausal Women.* [online] Available at: https://www.ncbi.nlm.nih.gov/pmc/articles/PMC4713270/ .

63 Harvard Health Publishing. (n.d.). Gum disease may signal warning for pancreatic cancer. https://www.health.harvard.edu/staying-healthy/gum-disease-may-signal-warning-for-pancreatic-cancer

64 Periodontology, A. (2019). Diabetes and Periodontal Disease | Perio.org. https://www.perio.org/consumer/gum-disease-and-diabetes.htm

65 Beck M. (2019). If Your Teeth Could Talk ... https://baledoneen.com/if-your-teeth-could-talk/

66 (2019). Retrieved from http://www.ginecologo-ostetrica.it/wp-content/uploads/2017/05/1_IgieneOrala_oral_health_during_pregnancy1.pdf

67 https://www.aafp.org/afp/2008/0415/p1139.html

About the Author

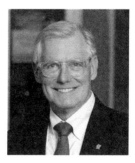

Dr. V Kim Kutsch DMD is a retired dentist of 40 years. He is a prolific writer, thought leader, inventor, and researcher in the field of dental caries and minimally invasive dentistry. He acts as a reviewer of the *Journal of the American Dental Association* and *Compendium*. Dr. Kutsch is the CEO and founder of Dental Alliance Holdings LLC, manufacturers of the CariFree system and is a Scientific Advisor of Dental Caries at the prestigious Kois Center. When he isn't writing, researching, or advising, Dr. Kutsch enjoys spending time with his wife Dana, his children, and grandchildren. He also enjoys fishing, painting, and playing the banjo.